Device Associated Infections

Guest Editor

PREETI N. MALANI, MD

INFECTIOUS DISEASE CLINICS OF NORTH AMERICA

www.id.theclinics.com

Consulting Editor
ROBERT C. MOELLERING Jr, MD

March 2012 • Volume 26 • Number 1

SAUNDERS an imprint of ELSEVIER, Inc.

W.B. SAUNDERS COMPANY

A Division of Elsevier Inc.

1600 John F. Kennedy Blvd., Suite 1800, Philadelphia, PA 19103-2899.

http://www.theclinics.com

INFECTIOUS DISEASE CLINICS OF NORTH AMERICA Volume 26, Number 1
March 2012 ISSN 0891–5520, ISBN-13: 978-1-4557-3879-3

Editor: Stephanie Donley
Developmental Editor: Teia Stone

Infectious Disease Clinics of North America (ISSN 0891–5520) is published in March, June, September, and December by Elsevier Inc., 360 Park Avenue South, New York, NY 10010-1710. Periodicals postage paid at New York, NY and additional mailing offices. Subscription prices are $271.00 per year for US individuals, $463.00 per year for US institutions, $134.00 per year for US students, $321.00 per year for Canadian individuals, $573.00 per year for Canadian institutions, $383.00 per year for international individuals, $573.00 per year for international institutions, and $185.00 per year for Canadian and international students. To receive student rate, orders must be accompanied by name of affiliated institution, date of term, and the *signature* of program/residency coordinator on institution letterhead. Orders will be billed at individual rate until proof of status is received. Foreign air speed delivery is included in all *Clinics* subscription prices. All prices are subject to change without notice. **POSTMASTER**: Send address changes to *Infectious Disease Clinics of North America,* Elsevier Health Sciences Division, Subcription Customer Service, 3251 Riverport Lane, Maryland Heights, MO 63043. **Customer Service: 1-800-654-2452 (US). From outside of the US and Canada, call 1-314-447-8871. Fax: 1-314-447-8029. E-mail: JournalsCustomerService-usa@elsevier.com (print support) or JournalsOnlineSupport-usa@elsevier.com (online support).**

Infectious Disease Clinics of North America is also published in Spanish by Editorial Inter-MÅdica, Junin 917, 1er A 1113, Buenos Aires, Argentina.

Reprints. For copies of 100 or more, of articles in this publication, please contact the Commercial Reprints Department, Elsevier Inc., 360 Park Avenue South, New York, New York 10010-1710. Tel. (212) 633-3812, Fax: (212) 462-1935, E-mail: reprints@elsevier.com.

Infectious Disease Clinics of North America is covered in *MEDLINE/PubMed (Index Medicus), Current Contents/ Clinical Medicine, Science Citation Alert, SCISEARCH,* and *Research Alert.*

Printed and bound by CPI Group (UK) Ltd, Croydon, CR0 4YY

Transferred to Digital Print 2012

Contributors

CONSULTING EDITOR

ROBERT C. MOELLERING Jr, MD
Shields Warren-Mallinckrodt Professor of Medical Research, Harvard Medical School; Department of Medicine, Beth Israel Deaconess Medical Center, Boston, Massachusetts

GUEST EDITOR

PREETI N. MALANI, MD, MSJ
Research Scientist, Associate Professor of Medicine, Divisions of Infectious Diseases and Geriatric Medicine, Department of Internal Medicine, University of Michigan Medical School, Ann Arbor Veterans Affairs Ann Arbor Healthcare System, Ann Arbor, Michigan

AUTHORS

WENDY S. ARMSTRONG, MD, FIDSA
Associate Professor of Medicine, Division of Infectious Disease, Emory University School of Medicine, Atlanta, Georgia

NATASHA BAGDASARIAN, MD, MPH
Assistant Professor of Medicine, Divisions of General Medicine and Infectious Diseases, University of Michigan and Veterans Affairs Ann Arbor Healthcare System, Ann Arbor, Michigan

SOPHIA CALIFANO, MD
Chief Medical Resident, Department of Internal Medicine, University of Michigan, Ann Arbor, Michigan

CAROL E. CHENOWETH, MD
Professor of Medicine, Division of Infectious Diseases; Hospital Epidemiologist, Department of Infection Control and Epidemiology, University of Michigan, Ann Arbor, Michigan

THOMAS CRAWFORD, MD
Clinical Assistant Professor of Medicine, Division of Cardiovascular Medicine, Cardiovascular Center, University of Michigan Medical School, Ann Arbor, Michigan

CHRISTOPHER J. CRNICH, MD, MS
Assistant Professor of Medicine, Division of Infectious Diseases, School of Medicine and Public Health, University of Wisconsin; Staff Physician and Hospital Epidemiologist, William S. Middleton Veterans Affairs Hospital, Madison, Wisconsin

PAUL DRINKA, MD
Clinical Professor, Division of Geriatrics, School of Medicine and Public Health, University of Wisconsin, Madison; Clinical Professor, Division of Geriatrics, Medical College of Wisconsin, Milwaukee; Department of Internal Medicine, School of Medicine and Public Health, University of Wisconsin, Medical College of Wisconsin, Milwaukee, Wisconsin

TEJAL GANDHI, MD
Clinical Assistant Professor of Medicine, Division of Infectious Diseases, University of Michigan Medical School, Ann Arbor, Michigan

KAROL GUTOWSKI, MD, FACS
Clinical Associate Professor, Division of Plastic Surgery, University of Chicago Pritzker School of Medicine, Chicago, Illinois

MICHAEL HEUNG, MD, MS
Assistant Professor of Medicine, Division of Nephrology, University of Michigan, Ann Arbor, Michigan

ANGELA L. HEWLETT, MD, MS
Assistant Professor of Internal Medicine, Division of Infectious Diseases, University of Nebraska Medical Center, Omaha, Nebraska

PREETI N. MALANI, MD, MSJ
Research Scientist, Associate Professor of Medicine, Division of Infectious Diseases and Geriatric Medicine, Veterans Affairs Ann Arbor Healthcare System, Geriatrics Research Education and Clinical Center (GRECC), University of Michigan, Ann Arbor, Michigan

LINDSAY E. NICOLLE, MD, FRCPC
Professor, Department of Internal Medicine and Medical Microbiology, University of Manitoba Health Sciences Centre, Winnipeg, Manitoba, Canada

FRANCIS D. PAGANI, MD, PhD
Otto Gago, M.D. Professor of Cardiac Surgery, Director, Surgical Director, Adult Heart Transplantation, Center for Circulatory Support, University of Michigan, Ann Arbor, Michigan

ROBIN PATEL, MD
Division of Clinical Microbiology, Department of Laboratory Medicine, and Pathology, Mayo Clinic; Division of Infectious Diseases, Department of Internal Medicine, Mayo Clinic, Rochester, Minnesota

JAMES RIDDELL IV, MD
Clinical Associate Professor of Medicine, Division of Infectious Diseases, University of Michigan Medical School, Ann Arbor, Michigan

MARK E. RUPP, MD
Professor of Internal Medicine, Division of Infectious Diseases; Medical Director, Department of Healthcare Epidemiology, University of Nebraska Medical Center, Omaha, Nebraska

EMILY K. SHUMAN, MD
Clinical Lecturer in Medicine, Division of Infectious Diseases, University of Michigan, Ann Arbor, Michigan

EDWARD STENEHJEM, MD
Fellow, Division of Infectious Diseases, Emory University School of Medicine, Atlanta, Georgia

GILBERT R. UPCHURCH Jr, MD
William H. Muller Jr. Professor of Surgery, Chief of Vascular and Endovascular Surgery, University of Virginia, Charlottesville, Virginia

ANDREW URQUHART, MD
Associate Professor, Department of Orthopaedic Surgery, University of Michigan, Ann Arbor, Michigan

PASCHALIS VERGIDIS, MD
Division of Clinical Microbiology, Department of Laboratory Medicine and Pathology, Mayo Clinic, Rochester, Minnesota

LARAINE L. WASHER, MD
Clinical Assistant Professor, Division of Infectious Diseases, Department of Internal Medicine; Associate Hospital Epidemiologist, Department of Infection Control and Epidemiology, University of Michigan Health System, Ann Arbor, Michigan

MICHAEL H. YOUNG, MD
Assistant Professor of Medicine, Division of Infectious Diseases, University of Kentucky School of Medicine, University of Kentucky, Lexington, Kentucky

Contents

Central line-associated bloodstream infections (CLA-BSI) are one of the leading causes of healthcare-associated infections, resulting in significant morbidity and substantial excess cost. There is a growing recognition that most CLA-BSIs are preventable. Elimination of preventable CLA-BSI is the focus of a recently released CDC Guideline. Universal preventative measures include collaborative performance improvement using checklists and bundles, education of persons who insert and maintain catheters, maximal sterile barrier precautions, and chlorhexidine skin preparation. Technologic innovations including coated catheters, antimicrobial impregnated dressings, and antimicrobial lock solutions should be considered if the rate of CLA-BSI is not acceptable after application of universal precautions.

Catheter-acquired urinary infection is the most common device-associated healthcare-acquired infection. Although most patients are asymptomatic, symptomatic infection may occur and is associated with increased morbidity and costs. Long-term indwelling catheters are associated with more complex microbiology and greater morbidity than short-term catheters. The most effective way to prevent these infections is to restrict indwelling urinary catheter use to limited indications, and to discontinue use of a catheter as soon as feasible. Alternate means of managing bladder emptying, including external condom catheters for men and intermittent catheterization for patients with neurologic impairment of bladder emptying, should be used when possible.

Prosthetic joint infection (PJI) is a serious complication of total joint arthroplasty (TJA) that can negatively affect functional status and quality of life. This article examines the epidemiology of PJI and reviews current diagnostic, treatment, and management strategies. Diagnosis can be challenging because presenting symptoms are often nonspecific and there is no simple gold standard diagnostic test. Successful treatment of PJI requires a combination of medical and surgical strategies. Given the devastating nature of PJI and the increasing numbers of TJAs performed, prevention efforts remain critical.

Infection after breast implant surgery occurs in 1.1% to 2.5% of procedures performed for augmentation and up to 35% of procedures performed for reconstruction after mastectomy. Most infections result from skin organisms and occur in the immediate postoperative period, although infections can occasionally present after many years. Diagnosis of breast implant infection relies on the clinical presentation of breast pain, swelling, erythema, and drainage in conjunction with ultrasound-guided cultures of periprosthetic fluid. Management commonly involves implant removal, with device salvage attempted in select situations.

Infectious complications remain a major source of morbidity and mortality for patients with end-stage renal disease on dialysis. The majority of these complications are related to dialysis access devices, and as such represent a potentially modifiable risk factor. This article reviews the important infectious complications associated with dialysis access, including both hemodialysis and peritoneal dialysis. The discussion highlights the epidemiology, management, and prevention of dialysis access infections.

Indwelling medical devices are increasingly used in long-term care facilities (LTCFs). These devices place residents at a heightened risk for infection and colonization and infection with multidrug-resistant organisms. Understanding the risk and pathogenesis of infection associated with commonly used medical devices can help facilitate appropriate therapy. Programs to minimize unnecessary use of indwelling medical devices in residents and maximize staff adherence to infection control and maintenance procedures are essential features of a LTCF infection prevention program. LTCFs that provide care for large numbers of residents with indwelling medical devices should routinely perform surveillance for device-related infections and develop systems for assessing the safety and efficacy of newly introduced device-related technology.

Reuse of both single-use and multiuse medical devices is a common practice and can result in transmission of infection when appropriate sterilization or reprocessing does not occur. Reuse of single-use devices can be problematic because there are no clear standards for reprocessing, although data regarding adverse outcomes are limited. Single-use devices are commonly reused, appropriately or inappropriately, in resource-limited settings because of cost constraints. Reuse of medical devices raises important legal and ethical questions.

The pathogenesis of device-associated infections is related to biofilm bacteria that exhibit distinct characteristics with respect to growth rate, structural features, and protection from host immune mechanisms and antimicrobial agents when compared with planktonic counterparts. Biofilm-associated infections are prevented, diagnosed, and treated differently from infections not associated with biofilms. This article reviews innovative concepts for the prevention of biofilm formation, and novel treatment approaches. Specific approaches for the diagnosis and prevention of catheter-associated urinary tract and bloodstream infections, as well as infections associated with orthopedic implants and cardiovascular implantable electronic devices, are also discussed.

VISIT THE CLINICS ONLINE!
Access your subscription at:
www.theclinics.com

Preface

Device-Associated Infections

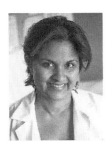

Preeti N. Malani, MD, MSJ
Guest Editor

Each year hundreds of thousands of patients undergo implantation of various medical devices, including prosthetic joints, urinary and venous catheters, and left ventricular assist devices. Although these technologies can improve quality and sometimes even quantity of life, infection remains a potentially devastating complication. Besides significant morbidity and functional impairment, device-associated infection presents a considerable economic burden, accounting for hundreds of millions of dollars in excess health care costs. Despite improved diagnostics and an expanding antimicrobial armamentarium, successful treatment of device-associated infection remains a vital clinical challenge.

From an infectious diseases standpoint, the most predictably effective approach to manage an infected device is to simply "take it out"; however, some devices cannot be easily removed and some patients are not candidates for additional operative procedures. Although treatment with antimicrobials alone is generally inadequate given the physiology of biofilms, long-term suppressive therapy can sometimes palliate symptoms. The need to strike a fine balance between the desire for clinical cure and the need to maintain physical function and quality of life is the very quintessence of device infection. These concerns are perhaps most critical among older adults, who receive a disproportionate number of devices and experience a larger number of infectious complications. As such, an ongoing discussion of the overall goals of care must be an integral part of every treatment plan.

Dramatic improvements in engineering and design help make device development one of the most dynamic fields in medicine. Thirty years ago, cardiac surgeons (not cardiologists) placed implantable cardioverter-defibrillators via thoracotomy; today cardiologists (not cardiac surgeons) can use a percutaneous approach to place short-term left ventricular assist devices. With rapidly evolving technology comes the need for infectious diseases specialists to maintain an understanding of the many technical nuances intrinsic to new devices.

Infect Dis Clin N Am 26 (2012) xiii–xiv
doi:10.1016/j.idc.2011.09.013
0891-5520/12/$ – see front matter © 2012 Elsevier Inc. All rights reserved.

id.theclinics.com

Optimal management of device-associated infections requires a collaborative approach among surgical and medical specialists—a need that is central to the current issue of *Infectious Diseases Clinics of North America*. This cooperative spirit is reflected in the authorship, which includes infectious diseases experts as well as authorities in surgical (vascular, orthopedic, plastics, and cardiac) and nonsurgical (nephrology, cardiology, geriatrics) specialties.

Collectively, this issue of the *Clinics* examines best practices for these complex infections. In addition to the epidemiology, management, and prevention of commonly encountered device-associated infections, each review offers technical background on specific devices and related operative procedures. Areas of ongoing investigation are highlighted, including innovative concepts for the prevention of biofilm formation and biofilm-directed therapeutics. Emerging issues related to reuse of medical devices in resource-limited settings are also considered.

As device use continues to burgeon, the role of the infectious disease consultant will remain indispensable. The authors and I hope that you find this issue of the *Clinics* to be a practical and up-to-date resource.

Preeti N. Malani, MD, MSJ
Department of Internal Medicine
Divisions of Infectious Diseases and Geriatric Medicine
University of Michigan and
Ann Arbor Veterans Affairs Ann Arbor Healthcare System
Geriatric Research Education and Clinical Center
2215 Fuller Road, 111-I, 8th Floor
Ann Arbor, MI 48105, USA

E-mail address:
pmalani@umich.edu

New Developments in the Prevention of Intravascular Catheter Associated Infections

Angela L. Hewlett, MD, MS[a],*, Mark E. Rupp, MD[a,b]

KEYWORDS

- Bloodstream infection • Central venous catheter
- Intravascular catheter • Catheter-related bloodstream infection

Central line–associated bloodstream infections (CLA-BSIs) are one of the leading causes of health care–associated infections (HAI). These infections result in significant morbidity along with excess health care costs. In the past, the majority of central venous catheters (CVCs) were used only in intensive care units (ICUs). Currently CVCs are present in multiple health care settings, including long-term care facilities, home health care, and outpatient hemodialysis centers.

There is a growing recognition that many CLA-BSIs are preventable through the use of existing technology and clinical practice techniques. The ubiquitous nature of these catheters, along with the attributable morbidity, mortality, and excess costs of CLA-BSI, has led to concerted infection-control efforts aimed at preventing CLA-BSIs. The epidemiology, pathogenesis, and new developments in the prevention of CLA-BSI are discussed here. The diagnosis and management of CLA-BSI are beyond the scope of this article, and have been recently reviewed.[1]

EPIDEMIOLOGY

The National Healthcare Safety Network (NHSN) collects data on the incidence of CLA-BSI in the United States. According to the NHSN data from 2006 to 2008, the

Dr Hewlett has no relevant conflicts of interest to disclose. Dr Rupp has received research funding from Arrow International, 3 M, Becton Dickinson, and Molnlycke. Dr Rupp has served as a consultant or received honoraria from 3 M, Baxter, Semprus, and Care Fusion.
[a] Division of Infectious Diseases, University of Nebraska Medical Center, 985400 Nebraska Medical Center, Omaha, NE 68198, USA
[b] Department of Healthcare Epidemiology, University of Nebraska Medical Center, 984031 Nebraska Medical Center, Omaha, NE 68198, USA
* Corresponding author.
E-mail address: alhewlett@unmc.edu

Infect Dis Clin N Am 26 (2012) 1–11
doi:10.1016/j.idc.2011.09.002
0891-5520/12/$ – see front matter © 2012 Elsevier Inc. All rights reserved.

risk of CLA-BSI varies by the type of ICU or inpatient setting. The pooled mean CLA-BSI rates from range from 0.8 per 1000 catheter-days (inpatient rehabilitation wards) to 5.5 per 1000 catheter-days (critical care burn units).[2] These rates relate to surveillance, and may overestimate the true incidence of CLA-BSI because all bloodstream infections do not originate from the CVC. However, the NHSN rates are risk adjusted, and are used by facilities for benchmarking of individual CLA-BSI rates. Other factors found to influence CLA-BSI rates are patient-related factors including severity of illness, catheter-related factors such as the type of catheter used and site of catheter placement, and institutional factors including the number of beds at the facility and academic affiliation.[3]

In 2001, the Centers for Disease Control and Prevention (CDC) estimated that 43,000 CLA-BSIs occurred in ICUs across the United States.[4] In 2009, the estimated number of CLA-BSIs in ICUs in the United States decreased to 18,000, representing a 58% decrease in ICU CLA-BSIs during a 9-year period. Along with a reduction in morbidity and mortality, this decrease also results in substantial cost savings because each CLA-BSI has been estimated to increase health care costs by $16,550.[4] These reductions are largely thought to be due to new developments in quality improvement and new technologies aimed at CLA-BSI prevention. However, it was noted that more CLA-BSIs occur in other inpatient and dialysis unit settings than in ICUs, and the total number of CLA-BSIs estimated to occur each year in United States ICUs, dialysis units, and inpatient units is 78,000.[4] Reliable surveillance data for CLA-BSIs in other care settings such as home care, long-term care, and long-term acute care are lacking, and the total number of CLA-BSIs in all care settings is undoubtedly substantial.

PATHOGENESIS

The pathogenesis of CLA-BSI involves interactions between the offending organism, the intravascular catheter, and the patient. Microbes most often gain access to short-term, nontunneled intravascular catheters via the patient's skin and migrate transcutaneously over the external surface of the catheter.[5] These organisms may stem from endogenous skin colonization or may result from extrinsic skin or catheter contamination. The longer an intravascular catheter remains in place, the more likely it is that aseptic practices are neglected and hub contamination occurs. Microorganisms then colonize the luminal surface of the catheter to result in a CLA-BSI. Although other routes of inoculation are thought to be involved less frequently, CLA-BSIs can also be caused by hematogenous seeding of the catheter from a distant site or by infusion of a contaminated substance. After encountering the intravascular catheter, the organisms subsequently adhere to the catheter, multiply, and produce biofilm. Biofilms are complex communities of microorganisms encased in a matrix consisting of polysaccharides, proteins, and nucleic acid derived from both the host and microbe.[6–8] Microorganisms existing in a mature biofilm-associated infection behave very differently to microorganisms growing in the planktonic state, and are generally less susceptible to antimicrobials and host immune response.[9] Infected intravascular catheters often must be removed for successful treatment.[10] **Fig. 1** illustrates the appearance of Staphylococcus aureus biofilm.

NEW DEVELOPMENTS

The recently released Healthcare Infection Control Practices Advisory Committee (HICPAC) Guidelines for the Prevention of Intravascular Catheter-Related Infections reinforce that programs to prevent CLA-BSI should be multidisciplinary.[3] Using performance improvement initiatives to decrease CLA-BSI rates by increasing compliance

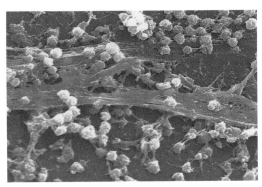

Fig. 1. Electron micrograph of *Staphylococcus aureus* biofilm. (*Courtesy of* CDC/Rodney M. Donlan, PhD, Janice Carr.)

with evidence-based practices is recommended in the new guidelines. Participants should include members the health care team: those who insert, remove, and maintain CVCs, infection control personnel, hospital administrators, and patients who are able to assist in catheter maintenance. Similar to the previous guidelines published in 2002, the new recommendations emphasize the education of health care workers as well as continuous assessment of knowledge and adherence to guidelines for those involved in insertion and maintenance of CVC.[11] The new guidelines also discuss the use of new technologies to aid in the reduction of CLA-BSI rates. The consensus of many experts is that introduction of technological advances may be necessary if implementation of performance improvement initiatives does not successfully minimize the incidence of CLA-BSI.

Updated and modified recommendations included in the new guidelines are outlined in **Table 1**.

PREVENTION: PERFORMANCE INITIATIVES

Alterations in clinical practice and educational interventions aimed at preventing HAIs through large-scale quality-improvement projects have gained recognition during the last decade. The Pittsburgh Regional Healthcare Initiative, instituted in 2001, used multiple infection control interventions in an effort to reduce CLA-BSI. Thirty-two hospitals in Pennsylvania participated in the project. Interventions included promotion of evidence-based catheter insertion practices and recording adherence to these practices, educational modules about CLA-BSI prevention, a standardized catheter insertion kit, and reporting CLA-BSI rates back to participating hospitals. Data analysis during the intervention period (April 2001 to March 2005) indicated that the pooled mean rate of CLA-BSI in the participating ICUs decreased by 68%.[12]

The Michigan Health and Hospital Association Keystone ICU Project is another large-scale quality-improvement initiative focused on reducing HAIs. The project involved a bundle of evidence-based interventions in an attempt to decrease the CLA-BSI rates. The interventions focused on appropriate hand hygiene, the use of chlorhexidine for skin preparation, the use of full-barrier precautions during insertion, the use of the subclavian vein as the preferred insertion site, and the removal of unnecessary CVCs. Data from 67 hospitals (103 ICUs) in Michigan were included. During the initial study period (March 2004 to September 2005), CLA-BSI rates decreased by 66%.[13] These results were sustained for an additional 18 months after completion of the study period.[14] Implementation of the Keystone Project was also associated

Table 1
Summary of updated recommendations from guidelines for the prevention of intravascular catheter-related infections (2011)

Subject	Recommendation
Placement of central venous catheters	Use ultrasound guidance to place central venous catheters (if this technology is available) to reduce the number of cannulation attempts and mechanical complications. Ultrasound guidance should only be used by those fully trained in its technique. (category IB)
Skin preparation	Prepare clean skin with a >0.5% chlorhexidine preparation with alcohol before central venous catheter and peripheral arterial catheter insertion and during dressing changes. If there is a contraindication to chlorhexidine, tincture of iodine, an iodophor, or 70% alcohol can be used as alternatives. (category IA)
Catheter site dressing regimens	Use a chlorhexidine-impregnated sponge dressing for temporary short-term catheters in patients older than 2 months of age if the CLABSI rate is not decreasing despite adherence to basic prevention measures, including education and training, appropriate use of chlorhexidine for skin antisepsis, and maximal sterile barrier precautions. (category IB)
Patient cleansing	Use a 2% chlorhexidine wash for daily skin cleansing to reduce CRBSI. (category II)
Catheter securement devices	Use a sutureless securement device to reduce the risk of infection for intravascular catheters (category II)
Antimicrobial lock solutions	Use prophylactic antimicrobial lock solution in patients with long-term catheters who have a history of multiple CRBSI despite optimal maximal adherence to aseptic technique. (category II)
Antimicrobial-impregnated central venous catheters	Use a chlorhexidine/silver sulfadiazine-impregnated or minocycline/rifampin-impregnated CVC in patients whose catheter is expected to remain in place >5 days if, after successful implementation of a comprehensive strategy to reduce rates of CLABSI, the CLABSI rate is not decreasing. The comprehensive strategy should include at least the following 3 components: educating persons who insert and maintain catheters, use of maximal sterile barrier precautions, and a >0.5% chlorhexidine preparation with alcohol for skin antisepsis during CVC insertion. (category IA)
Needleless intravascular catheter systems	Use a needleless system to access IV tubing. (category IC) When needleless systems are used, a split septum valve may be preferred over some mechanical valves, due to increased risk of infection with the mechanical valves. (category II)
Performance improvement	Use hospital-specific or collaborative-based performance improvement initiatives in which multifaceted strategies are "bundled" together to improve compliance with evidence-based recommended practices. (category IB)

Level of evidence for recommendations: category IA, strongly recommended for implementation and strongly supported by well-designed experimental, clinical, or epidemiologic studies; category IB, strongly recommended for implementation and supported by some experimental, clinical, or epidemiologic studies and a strong theoretical rationale; or an accepted practice (eg, aseptic technique) supported by limited evidence; category IC, required by state or federal regulations, rules, or standards; category II, suggested for implementation, and supported by suggestive clinical or epidemiologic studies or a theoretical rationale.

Abbreviations: CLABSI, central line–associated bloodstream infection; CRBSI, catheter-related bloodstream infection; CVC, central venous catheter.

Data from O'Grady NP, Alexander M, Burns LA, et al. Guidelines for the prevention of intravascular catheter-related infections. Clin Infect Dis 2011;52(9):e162–93.

with a statistically significant decrease in hospital mortality in Michigan.[15] The results of this initiative further affirmed that bundled infection control interventions can result in a marked reduction in CLA-BSI. However, important unanswered questions remain with this approach regarding levels of compliance with bundle recommendations, the relative importance of bundle elements, validation of surveillance data, and the role of technologic innovations and devices.

The HICPAC guidelines suggest the use of collaborative performance improvement initiatives that use bundles of interventions to improve compliance with evidence-based recommended practices.[3] Comprehensive strategies should include education of those who insert and maintain CVCs, using a greater than 0.5% chlorhexidine preparation with alcohol for skin antisepsis during CVC insertion, and using maximal sterile barrier precautions.

The new guidelines also emphasize that only trained personnel who demonstrate competence in CVC insertion and maintenance should be assigned these tasks, and that periodic assessment of these individuals should occur. A stronger statement is included regarding the importance of ensuring appropriate nursing staff levels in ICUs, because elevated patient-to-nurse ratios have been associated with the occurrence of CLA-BSI.[16]

PREVENTION: TECHNOLOGIC INNOVATIONS

The use of new technologies as methods to prevent CLA-BSI has also come to the forefront, and is emphasized in the new HICPAC guidelines. Ultrasound guidance, antimicrobial and antiseptic-impregnated CVCs, chlorhexidine washes, antiseptic-impregnated catheter dressings, and anti-infective lock solutions have all been used in multiple studies with substantial degrees of success.

The use of ultrasound guidance to place CVCs is a relatively new practice. In the hands of an experienced operator, the use of real-time ultrasound guidance has been shown to decrease mechanical complications and reduce the number of cannulation attempts when compared with CVC placement using anatomic landmarks alone.[17–20] A meta-analysis of 18 trials demonstrated that the use of ultrasound guidance decreased the number of failed catheterization attempts, catheter placement complications, failures on the first attempt, attempts to successful catheterization, and the time to successful catheterization. This benefit was seen over a wide range of operator experience and in various settings.[18] The use of ultrasound guidance is an attractive tool to reduce the incidence of mechanical complications so as to make CVC insertion a safer practice.

Although chlorhexidine-based skin preparations were recommended in the previous HICPAC guideline, the amount of chlorhexidine present in the preparation that is necessary to prevent CLA-BSI was decreased to 0.5% in the new recommendations. This guideline was secondary to the emergence of data indicating that less potent chlorhexidine concentrations were equally as effective, better tolerated, and induced fewer skin reactions. Another addition was the recommendation of alcohol-containing chlorhexidine solutions, because the use of these preparations demonstrated a statistically significant decrease in CLA-BSI in several studies.[21] However, it should be noted that there are no data comparing skin preparation with solutions containing chlorhexidine and alcohol with those containing povidone-iodine and alcohol. This area is one that deserves further study to delineate whether the observed decrease in CLA-BSI rates was attributable to the presence of chlorhexidine or the presence of alcohol.

No recommendation is made regarding the use of chlorhexidine for skin preparation in neonates aged less than 2 months, and chlorhexidine is not currently approved by the Food and Drug Administration for use in this population, due to lack of evidence for its safety and efficacy. However, according to a recent survey, chlorhexidine use in neonates is a common practice, with 59% of survey respondents reporting the use of chlorhexidine for CVC insertion in their Neonatal Intensive Care Unit (NICU).[22] Most NICUs are further qualifying the use of chlorhexidine based on gestational age, birth weight, or chronologic age.[22]

The new HICPAC guideline also adds a recommendation to consider use of chlorhexidine-impregnated sponge dressings with temporary short-term catheters in patients older than 2 months if, despite concerted prevention efforts, the CLA-BSI rate is not decreasing. Several studies, including a large multicenter randomized controlled trial, have demonstrated a reduction in CLA-BSI rates when chlorhexidine-impregnated sponge dressings were used instead of standard dressings in ICU patients.[23,24] It must be noted that this multicenter trial was conducted in France before chlorhexidine skin preparations had become commercially available, thus it is unclear as to whether the use of chlorhexidine for routine skin preparation would have influenced the outcome of the study, either by muting the effect of the chlorhexidine sponge dressings or further decreasing CLA-BSI rates. There are insufficient data to recommend the use of chlorhexidine-impregnated sponge dressings in long-term catheters such as tunneled dialysis catheters or peripherally inserted central venous catheter (PICC) lines.[3] Other forms of chlorhexidine-impregnated dressings are commercially available, but clinical data regarding prevention of CLA-BSI remains lacking and thus no recommendations are made for their use.

The use of a chlorhexidine/silver sulfadiazine-impregnated or minocycline/rifampin-impregnated CVC is suggested in patients whose catheter is expected to remain in place longer than 5 days if, after successful implementation of a comprehensive strategy to reduce rates of CLA-BSI, the CLA-BSI rate is not decreasing.[3] This recommendation is not necessarily a new one, because the previous guidelines recommended the use of coated catheters if the CLA-BSI rate remained above the goal set by the institution.[11] First-generation chlorhexidine/silver sulfadiazine catheters were shown to reduce the risk of CLA-BSI when compared with standard noncoated catheters.[25] A newer, second-generation version of this catheter is coated with chlorhexidine on the internal surface and a higher concentration of chlorhexidine/silver sulfadiazine on the external luminal surface. Catheters impregnated with minocycline/rifampin have also been shown to reduce the CLA-BSI rates compared with first-generation chlorhexidine/silver sulfadiazine catheters and with noncoated catheters.[26,27] Limited data comparing minocycline/rifampin-impregnated catheters to second-generation chlorhexidine/silver sulfadiazine-impregnated catheters are available. Comparative studies of this nature are necessary for recommending the use of one type of coated catheter over another, and should be the focus of further research efforts. There is some concern that antimicrobial-impregnated catheters may lead to increased antimicrobial resistance. However, in carefully monitored studies conducted over multiple years, rifampin or minocycline resistance has not been observed.[28] Therefore, catheters coated with either chlorhexidine/silver sulfadiazine or minocycline/rifampin are effective in preventing microbial colonization and bloodstream infection, whereas data are lacking regarding catheters coated with other agents such as carbon/platinum/silver, benzalkonium chloride, or miconazole/rifampin.

The components of the comprehensive strategy that should be implemented before using coated catheters routinely are detailed, and include education of the operator, the use of maximal sterile barrier precautions during catheter insertion, and the use of 0.5% chlorhexidine with alcohol for skin preparation. In the face of decreasing rates of CLA-BSI due to other interventions, studies demonstrating that the use of coated catheters produces a statistically significant further reduction in CLA-BSI may be difficult.

The new guidelines give a stronger recommendation for the use of antimicrobial lock solutions for prevention of CLA-BSI. This technique involves filling a catheter lumen with an antimicrobial solution and allowing it to remain in place while the catheter is not in use. The use of antimicrobial lock solutions is suggested in patients with long-term CVCs who have recurrent CLA-BSIs despite optimal adherence to aseptic technique. This recommendation is based on data that demonstrated a reduction in CLA-BSI in selected patient populations requiring long-term catheters. These studies involved patients generally considered to be at high risk for CLA-BSI, and included dialysis patients, intestinal failure patients on long-term parenteral nutrition, and oncology patients receiving chemotherapy. The studies used antibiotic lock solutions as well as nonantibiotic lock solutions such as ethanol and recombinant tissue plasminogen activator (rt-PA).[29–31] Studies on novel lock solutions are also promising, and warrant further investigation.[32]

Using a 2% chlorhexidine wash for daily skin cleansing is also suggested as a method to reduce CLA-BSI.[3] This relatively simple strategy has been used in several studies, including a large single-center study that demonstrated that ICU patients bathed in chlorhexidine were significantly less likely to acquire a primary bloodstream infection than those bathed with soap and water.[33,34] Routine chlorhexidine bathing has been primarily studied in ICUs, although one study demonstrated a decrease in CLA-BSI by implementing routine chlorhexidine bathing in a long-term acute-care hospital.[35] Chlorhexidine bathing has been studied in general medical wards for prevention of HAIs, but an effect on CLA-BSI rates has not been conclusively demonstrated.[36] Further studies are under way in non-ICU patients, which will determine whether routine chlorhexidine bathing is appropriate in other settings and patient populations. Of note, in most of the studies involving the introduction of chlorhexidine bathing the baseline CLA-BSI rates were relatively high, so it is unclear whether this effect will be readily seen in facilities with low baseline rates of CLA-BSI.

Other changes in the new guidelines involve the use of needleless systems, which are now ubiquitous in the health care environment. Needleless systems were originally designed to reduce the frequency of needle-stick injuries by health care workers, thus reducing exposure to blood-borne pathogens. Despite these safety benefits, multiple reports of increasing CLA-BSI rates as a result of introduction of needleless connectors are appearing.[37–39] One in vitro study demonstrated that needleless connectors readily acquire biofilm formation, which may contribute to the incidence of CLA-BSI.[40] Appropriate disinfection of the connector surfaces is thought to be an important component in reducing the risk of CLA-BSI when needleless systems are used. However, it is not clear whether one disinfectant is superior to another for this application, nor is it known how long the connector hubs should be scrubbed. There is also potential for the usage of antimicrobial connectors to decrease the likelihood of microbial contamination of the needleless system, and this novel technology deserves further study.[40]

Previously listed as an unresolved issue, the use of sutureless securement devices for intravascular catheters is now recommended as a category II (limited data) recommendation. Use of these devices may decrease catheter colonization by maintaining the integrity of the surrounding tissues, which may be an important element in reducing CLA-BSI.[41]

SUMMARY

Results like those from the Pittsburgh Regional Healthcare Initiative and the Michigan Keystone Project have confirmed that many CLA-BSIs are preventable, and have led to an expectation that drastic reduction of CLA-BSI will be achieved. The Centers for Medicaid and Medicare Services no longer reimburses hospitals for excess costs associated with CLA-BSI.[42] Many states now require public reporting of hospital-specific CLA-BSI rates.[43] As a result of the American Recovery and Reinvestment Act of 2009, the CDC provided $40 million to state health departments to fund promotion of HAI prevention programs.[4] State health departments are working with health care facility partners, state hospital associations, and various quality-improvement organizations to implement initiatives targeted at HAI prevention. National quality-improvement programs like the Comprehensive Unit-Based Safety Program from the Agency for Healthcare Research and Quality in partnership with the American Hospital Association and Johns Hopkins University seek to improve the culture of patient safety as well as replicate the success of the Keystone Project in reducing CLA-BSI. Participating hospitals agree to implement a checklist to ensure compliance with safety practices, educate staff on evidence-based practices to reduce CLA-BSIs, educate staff on team training, provide feedback on infection rates to hospitals and hospital units, and implement monthly team meetings to assess progress.

Although the data on decreasing CLA-BSI rates in the ICU setting is encouraging, CVCs are used in a wide variety of other health care settings that deserve attention. CVCs are increasingly used in the outpatient setting as well as in long-term care facilities. PICCs are widely used to provide long-term intravenous access. PICCs are used in the outpatient setting, and are often supplanting conventional CVCs in the inpatient setting.[44] These catheters are placed for multiple indications, including hemodialysis, chemotherapy, total parenteral nutrition, anti-infective therapy, and transfusion therapy. The coordinated efforts to improve CLA-BSI rates in ICUs may not necessarily be effective in non-ICU settings, and the increasing use of different types of CVCs in various environments necessitates further research on methods of CLA-BSI prevention.

It is now thought that many, if not the vast majority, of CLA-BSIs are potentially preventable. Elimination of preventable CLA-BSI through multifaceted prevention strategies is the focus of the new HICPAC guidelines. As baseline CLA-BSI rates continue to decrease through the use of multiple preventive measures, it is becoming increasingly difficult to demonstrate the effects of individual interventions on CLA-BSI rates. However, the effects of these interventions may still be seen in patient populations that are at high risk for CLA-BSI, and this is where further study should be targeted. Because most of these new performance initiatives and technologies focus on the initial insertion of CVCs, research efforts should be directed to the ongoing care and maintenance of catheters to continue to improve clinical practice and decrease central line–associated infections.

Although many studies have influenced the recommendations in the HICPAC Guidelines for the Prevention of Intravascular Catheter-Related Infections, many unanswered questions remain. Of note, several of the new recommendations in the guidelines have only a category II level of evidence, meaning that they are suggested for implementation and are supported by suggestive clinical or epidemiologic studies or a theoretical rationale. Further studies are necessary in order to support these and other recommendations and to fill the gaps in knowledge on the best methods to prevent CLA-BSI. As additional data are accrued, clinical practice and practice guidelines should keep pace and be adjusted accordingly.

REFERENCES

1. Weber DJ, Rutala WA. Central line-associated bloodstream infections: prevention and management. Infect Dis Clin North Am 2011;25(1):77–102.

2. Edwards JR, Peterson KD, Banerjee S, et al. National Healthcare Safety Network (NHSN) report: data for 2006 through 2008, issued December 2009. Am J Infect Control 2009;37:783–805.
3. O'Grady NP, Alexander M, Burns LA, et al. Guidelines for the prevention of intravascular catheter-related infections. Clin Infect Dis 2011;52(9):e162–93.
4. Centers for Disease Control and Prevention (CDC). Vital signs: central line-associated blood stream infections—United States, 2001, 2008, and 2009. MMWR Morb Mortal Wkly Rep 2011;60(8):243–8.
5. Yanagi H, Sherertz RJ. Infections of intravascular catheters and vascular devices. In: Crossley KB, Jefferson KK, Archer G, et al, editors. Staphylococci in human disease. 2nd edition. Chichester, West Sussex: Wiley-Blackwell; 2009. p. 363–77.
6. Petri WA Jr, Mann BJ, Huston CD. Microbial adherence. In: Mandell GL, Bennett JE, Douglas RG Jr, editors. Principles and practice of infectious diseases'. 7th edition. Philadelphia: Churchill Livingstone Elsevier; 2009. p. 15–25.
7. Donlan RM, Costerton JW. Biofilms: survival mechanisms of clinically relevant microorganisms. Clin Microbiol Rev 2002;15:167–93.
8. Fey PD, Olson ME. Current concepts in biofilm formation of *Staphylococcus epidermidis*. Future Microbiol 2010;5:917–33.
9. Lewis K, Spoering AL, Kaldalu N, et al. Persiters: specialized cells responsible for biofilm tolerance. In: Pace JL, Rupp ME, Finch RG, editors. Biofilms, infection, and antimicrobial therapy. Boca Raton (FL): Taylor & Francis; 2006. p. 241–56.
10. Mermel LA, Allon M, Bouza E, et al. Clinical practice guidelines for the diagnosis and management of intravascular catheter-related infection: 2009 update by the infectious diseases society of America. Clin Infect Dis 2009;49:1–45.
11. O'Grady NP, Alexander M, Dellinger EP, et al. Guidelines for the prevention of intravascular catheter-related infections. Infect Control Hosp Epidemiol 2002; 23(12):759–69.
12. Centers for Disease Control and Prevention (CDC). Reduction in central line-associated bloodstream infections among patients in intensive care units—Pennsylvania, April 2001-March 2005. MMWR Morb Mortal Wkly Rep 2005;54(40): 1013–6.
13. Pronovost P, Needham D, Berenholtz S, et al. An intervention to decrease catheter-related bloodstream infections in the ICU. N Engl J Med 2006;355(26): 2725–32.
14. Pronovost PJ, Goeschel CA, Colantuoni E, et al. Sustaining reductions in catheter related bloodstream infections in Michigan intensive care units: observational study. BMJ 2010;340:c309.
15. Lipitz-Snyderman A, Steinwachs D, Needham DM, et al. Impact of a statewide intensive care unit quality improvement initiative on hospital mortality and length of stay: retrospective comparative analysis. BMJ 2011;342:d219.
16. Fridkin SK, Pear SM, Williamson TH, et al. The role of understaffing in central venous catheter-associated bloodstream infections. Infect Control Hosp Epidemiol 1996;17(3):150–8.
17. Froehlich CD, Rigby MR, Rosenberg ES, et al. Ultrasound-guided central venous catheter placement decreases complications and decreases placement attempts compared with the landmark technique in patients in a pediatric intensive care unit. Crit Care Med 2009;37(3):1090–6.
18. Hind D, Calvert N, McWilliams R, et al. Ultrasonic locating devices for central venous cannulation: meta-analysis. BMJ 2003;327(7411):361.

19. Randolph AG, Cook DJ, Gonzales CA, et al. Ultrasound guidance for placement of central venous catheters: a meta-analysis of the literature. Crit Care Med 1996; 24(12):2053–8.

20. Fragou M, Gravvanis A, Dimitriou V, et al. Real-time ultrasound-guided subclavian vein cannulation versus the landmark method in critical care patients: a prospective randomized study. Crit Care Med 2011;39(7):1607–12.

21. Chaiyakunapruk N, Veenstra DL, Lipsky BA, et al. Chlorhexidine compared with povidone-iodine solution for vascular catheter-site care: a meta-analysis. Ann Intern Med 2002;136(11):792–801.

22. Bryant KA, Zerr DM, Huskins WC, et al. The past, present, and future of health-care-associated infection prevention in pediatrics: catheter-associated bloodstream infections. Infect Control Hosp Epidemiol 2010;31(Suppl 1):S27–31.

23. Ruschulte H, Franke M, Gastmeier P, et al. Prevention of central venous catheter related infections with chlorhexidine gluconate impregnated wound dressings: a randomized controlled trial. Ann Hematol 2009;88(3):267–72.

24. Timsit JF, Schwebel C, Bouadma L, et al. Chlorhexidine-impregnated sponges and less frequent dressing changes for prevention of catheter-related infections in critically ill adults: a randomized controlled trial. JAMA 2009;301(12): 1231–41.

25. Veenstra DL, Saint S, Saha S, et al. Efficacy of antiseptic-impregnated central venous catheters in preventing catheter-related bloodstream infection: a meta-analysis. JAMA 1999;281:261–7.

26. Darouiche RO, Raad II, Heard SO, et al. A comparison of two antimicrobial-impregnated central venous catheters. Catheter Study Group. N Engl J Med 1999;340:1–8.

27. Raad I, Darouiche R, Dupuis J, et al. Central venous catheters coated with minocycline and rifampin for the prevention of catheter-related colonization and bloodstream infections. A randomized, double-blind trial. The Texas Medical Center Catheter Study Group. Ann Intern Med 1997;127:267–74.

28. Ramos ER, Reitzel R, Jiang Y, et al. Clinical effectiveness and risk of emerging resistance associated with prolonged use of antibiotic-impregnated catheters: more than 0.5 million catheter days and 7 years of clinical experience. Crit Care Med 2011;39(2):245–51.

29. Cober MP. Ethanol-lock therapy for the prevention of central venous access device infections in pediatric patients with intestinal failure. JPEN J Parenter Enteral Nutr 2011;35(1):67.

30. Hemmelgarn BR. Prevention of dialysis catheter malfunction with recombinant tissue plasminogen activator. N Engl J Med 2011;364(4):303.

31. Sanders J. A prospective double-blind randomized trial comparing intraluminal ethanol with heparinized saline for the prevention of catheter-associated bloodstream infection in immunosuppressed haematology patients. J Antimicrob Chemother 2008;62(4):809.

32. Maki DG, Ash SR, Winger RK, et al. A novel antimicrobial and antithrombotic lock solution for hemodialysis catheters: a multi-center, controlled, randomized trial. Crit Care Med 2011;39(4):613.

33. Bleasdale SC. Effectiveness of chlorhexidine bathing to reduce catheter-associated bloodstream infections in medical intensive care unit patients. Arch Intern Med 2007;167(19):2073.

34. Popovich KJ. Effectiveness of routine patient cleansing with chlorhexidine gluconate for infection prevention in the medical intensive care unit. Infect Control Hosp Epidemiol 2009;30(10):959.

35. Munoz-Price LS. Prevention of bloodstream infections by use of daily chlorhexidine baths for patients at a long-term acute care hospital. Infect Control Hosp Epidemiol 2009;30(11):1031.

36. Kassakian SZ, Mermel LA, Jefferson JA, et al. Impact of chlorhexidine bathing on hospital-acquired infections among general medical patients. Infect Control Hosp Epidemiol 2011;32(3):238–43.

37. Salgado CD, Chinnes L, Paczesny TH, et al. Increased rate of catheter-related bloodstream infection associated with use of a needleless mechanical valve device at a long-term acute care hospital. Infect Control Hosp Epidemiol 2007; 28(6):684–8.

38. Jarvis WR, Murphy C, Hall KK, et al. Health care-associated bloodstream infections associated with negative- or positive-pressure or displacement mechanical valve needleless connectors. Clin Infect Dis 2009;49(12):1821–7.

39. Rupp ME, Sholtz LA, Jourdan DR, et al. Outbreak of bloodstream infection temporally associated with the use of an intravascular needleless valve. Clin Infect Dis 2007;44(11):1408–14.

40. Maki DG. In vitro studies of a novel antimicrobial luer-activated needleless connector for prevention of catheter-related bloodstream infection. Clin Infect Dis 2010;50(12):1580.

41. Yamamoto AJ, Solomon JA, Soulen MC, et al. Sutureless securement device reduces complications of peripherally inserted central venous catheters. J Vasc Interv Radiol 2002;13(1):77–81.

42. Centers for Medicare and Medicaid Services. Hospital-acquired conditions. Available at: http://www.cms.gov/HospitalAcqCond/06_Hospital-Acquired_Conditions. asp. Accessed April 25, 2011.

43. McKibben L, Horan T, Tokars JI, et al. Guidance on public reporting of healthcare-associated infections: recommendations of the Healthcare Infection Control Practices Advisory Committee. Am J Infect Control 2005;33(4):217–26.

44. Safdar N, Maki DG. Risk of catheter-related bloodstream infection with peripherally inserted central venous catheters used in hospitalized patients. Chest 2005; 128(2):489–95.

Urinary Catheter-Associated Infections

Lindsay E. Nicolle, MD

KEYWORDS

- Urinary catheter • Urinary tract infection • Intermittent catheter
- Bacteriuria

The urinary catheter is one of the most common invasive devices used in health care. From 12% to 16% of acute-care inpatients have an indwelling urethral catheter inserted at some time during hospitalization, including 100% of patients undergoing selected surgical procedures and most patients admitted to critical care units.[1,2] A chronic indwelling catheter is present in about 5% of residents of long-term care facilities.[3] Intermittent catheterization is widely used for bladder emptying by individuals with spinal cord injury and other patients with neurologic impairment. This article addresses primarily the indwelling urethral catheter, and also discusses selected aspects relevant to intermittent catheterization. Other indwelling urinary devices, including ureteric stents and nephrostomy tubes, are not discussed.

Catheter-acquired urinary infection is an important problem in all healthcare settings. Infection of the urinary tract is one the most common healthcare-acquired infections, and 80% of these infections are attributed to an indwelling urinary catheter.[1,4] The costs of catheter-acquired urinary infection in acute-care hospitals are modest compared with other device-associated infections, such as central line bacteremia or ventilator-associated pneumonia, but the large number of patients with indwelling urinary catheters results in a substantial burden of morbidity and cost.[4] In addition, catheter-acquired urinary infection is the most common source of bacteremia in long-term care facilities, and symptomatic urinary infection is the most frequent infection experienced by spinal cord–injured patients managed with intermittent catheterization.[4] The urine drainage bag colonized with bacteria is also an important and ubiquitous environmental reservoir for resistant organisms in healthcare settings.[1]

DEFINITIONS

Urinary infection is catheter acquired if it develops while a urinary catheter is in situ or within 72 hours after device removal.[4] These infections are usually asymptomatic, and

The author has nothing to disclose.
Department of Internal Medicine and Medical Microbiology, University of Manitoba Health Sciences Centre, Room GG443 – 820, Sherbrook Street, Winnipeg, MB R3A 1R9, Canada
E-mail address: lnicolle@hsc.mb.ca

diagnosed when bacteria or yeast are isolated in appropriate quantitative counts from urine in the absence of clinical signs or symptoms attributed to the urinary tract. This is also referred to as "catheter-acquired bacteriuria." Symptomatic infection is diagnosed when there is bacteriuria associated with clinical signs and symptoms attributed to urinary infection. An indwelling urethral catheter is considered a short-term catheter when it remains in situ for less than 30 days and a long-term, or chronic, catheter when present 30 days or more. In-and-out catheterization is a single episode of catheterization with the catheter not retained in the bladder, and is usually performed for bladder emptying, volume measurement, or to obtain a urine specimen. Intermittent catheterization is the repeated use of an in-and-out catheter for bladder emptying, often performed by the individual themselves.

PATHOGENESIS
Bacteriuria

A urethral catheter facilitates entry of bacteria or yeast into the bladder through several mechanisms.[4,5] The most common route is ascension of bacterial biofilm along the tubing and catheter, with acquisition of bladder bacteriuria correlated with duration of catheterization.[6] In addition, periurethral organisms may be inoculated into the bladder at catheter insertion and, if the organism persists, bacteriuria is established. This is the usual means of acquisition of bacteriuria after intermittent catheterization or an in-and-out catheterization, but contributes to only a small proportion of early onset episodes of bacteriuria after insertion of an indwelling catheter. When an indwelling catheter is not managed appropriately, contaminated urine from the drainage bag or tubing may reflux into the bladder, or organisms may be introduced when there are breaks in the closed drainage system. The bulb of the indwelling catheter prevents complete bladder drainage, and a residual pool of undrained urine remains in the bladder. Organisms, once introduced, persist in this pool of urine, and in biofilm on the catheter or the bladder wall.

Biofilm is an inevitable consequence of indwelling catheter use. Immediately after insertion of the indwelling catheter, host proteins adhere to the catheter surface, forming a "conditioning layer."[5] This layer facilitates adherence of microorganisms that originate from the periurethral flora or are inoculated into the bag or drainage tube when these are manipulated. Once attached to the catheter surface, bacteria produce an exopolysaccharide coating within which bacterial colonies develop and persist. The biofilm also incorporates urinary components, such as Tamm-Horsfall protein and magnesium and calcium ions. Colonies of organisms within the biofilm exist in a protected environment that limits access to the bacteria by antibiotics or host defenses, such as neutrophils or immunoglobulins. Organisms are continually shed from the biofilm as daughter cells or biofilm aggregates and seed other sections of the catheter and the bladder. Biofilm ascends both the inside and outside surfaces of the catheter, and bladder bacteriuria is usually established within 1 or 2 weeks of catheter insertion.

The microbiology of the biofilm on the catheter and in bladder urine is dynamic. As long as the catheter remains in situ new organisms are continually incorporated into the biofilm and enter the bladder, while existing organisms are replaced. Some urease-producing organisms, such as *Proteus mirabilis* and *Providencia stuartii*, produce a greater amount of biofilm and this more rapidly ascends into the bladder. Hydrolysis of urea in the urine by urease-producing organisms such as these creates an alkaline environment favoring precipitation of magnesium and calcium ions to form a crystalline biofilm.[5] This material is similar to bladder and renal infection stones and may cause catheter encrustation and obstruction.[7]

Symptomatic Infection

The determinants of symptomatic catheter-acquired urinary tract infection are not well described. Catheter obstruction and trauma associated with mucosal bleeding are recognized associations preceding fever or bacteremia from a urinary source, but the proportion of symptomatic episodes attributed to these events is small. In a long-term care population, only 6 (8.1%) of 74 episodes of fever of presumed urinary origin were temporally associated with obstruction,[8] whereas a prospective study of men with chronic indwelling catheters reported the incidence of symptomatic urinary infection was similar for patients with or without episodes of catheter obstruction.[9] *Escherichia coli* isolates from the blood presumed to be of urinary origin in patients with an indwelling urethral catheter have fewer virulence factors compared with bacteremic strains isolated from patients with uncomplicated (non–catheter-related) urinary infection.[5,10] Strains isolated from patients with asymptomatic bacteriuria, with or without indwelling catheters, display a similar attenuation of *E coli* virulence determinants.[11] Thus, bacterial virulence does not play a pivotal role in the development of symptomatic infection. For subjects managed with intermittent catheterization, increased bladder pressure is an important risk factor for symptomatic infection. Other associations reported for women managed with intermittent catheterization are younger age and high catheterization volume and, for men, younger age, neurogenic bladder dysfunction especially with bladder leaking, and catheterization by someone other than the patient himself.[12]

Microbiology

The initial infection after insertion of a short-term catheter is usually with a single organism, most often *E coli* or other Enterobacteriaceae.[13,14] Yeast species, *Enterococcus* spp., and *Pseudomonas aeruginosa* may also occur. When there is a chronic indwelling catheter, on average three to five organisms are isolated from the urine at any time, including a wide variety of Enterobacteriaceae and other gram-negative organisms, gram-positive organisms, and yeast.[4] Urease-producing organisms, such as *P mirabilis*, *Klebsiella pneumoniae*, *Morganella morganii*, and *P stuartii*, are common.[15,16] *Candida albicans* is the most common yeast, but *C glabrata*, *C tropicalis*, and others also occur. Gram-positive organisms, such as coagulase-negative staphylococci and enterococcus species, are isolated frequently, but are less likely to be associated with symptomatic infection. Group B streptococcus and *Staphylococcus aureus* are relatively infrequent. Bacterial isolates from patients with catheter-acquired urinary infection are characterized by increased antimicrobial resistance. This is mainly attributed to prior healthcare exposures, including repeated antimicrobial courses for urinary tract or other infections. Vancomycin-resistant enterococcus and extended-spectrum β-lactamase–producing Enterobacteriaceae in acute-care hospitals and long-term care facilities are most frequently isolated from the urine of patients with indwelling catheters.

EPIDEMIOLOGY
Asymptomatic Bacteriuria

The rate of acquisition of bacteriuria is 3% to 7% per day for the patient with an indwelling catheter.[1,4] It is higher for women, for patients with increased periurethral colonization with potential uropathogens, and when there have been breaks in the closed drainage system within the previous 24 hours.[4] Patients receiving antimicrobial therapy have a lower rate of acquisition only for the first 4 days of catheterization. Patients with a chronic indwelling catheter have a prevalence of bacteriuria or funguria of 100%, but the incidence of acquisition of new organisms remains 3% to 7% per day. Some urease-producing organisms, such as *P mirabilis*, *K pneumonia*, and *P stuartii*, are more likely to persist, whereas such organisms as *Enterococcus* spp. resolve more rapidly.[15]

Bacteriuria is acquired after 3% to 5% of episodes of in-and-out catheterization. The prevalence of bacteriuria in spinal cord–injured patients managed with intermittent catheterization is 50%, and similar for men and women. These individuals experience an average of 18 to 24 episodes of new bacteriuria per person-year.[4] Infection is usually with a single organism, with *E coli* the most frequent species isolated.

Symptomatic Urinary Tract Infection

Symptomatic catheter-acquired urinary tract infection is uncommon in patients with short-term indwelling catheters despite widespread catheter use and the inevitable acquisition of bacteriuria with increasing duration of catheter use. A prospective study of 1497 acute-care patients after insertion of a new short-term catheter reported no difference in symptoms potentially attributable to urinary infection including fever, dysuria, urgency, or flank pain, for patients with or without bacteriuria.[13] Only four episodes of bacteremia (0.3% of catheters and 1.7% of bacteriuric catheters) had concordant blood and urine isolates, and only one of these had no potential source for bacteremia other than the urinary tract. A prospective randomized study comparing two different types of catheters reported an incidence of presumed symptomatic urinary infection of 1.43 to 1.61 per 100 indwelling catheter-days, and concordance of blood and urine isolates for bacteremic patients for only 0.52% of catheters placed and 4.8% of catheters with bacteriuria.[14] In critical care units, less than 3% of bacteremic episodes are attributed to catheter-acquired urinary infection.[4]

Episodes of fever occur more frequently in long-term care facility residents with indwelling catheters than those without, with this excess febrile morbidity attributed to urinary infection. More than 50% of episodes of fever in individuals with chronic indwelling catheters are from a urinary source, with an incidence of 0.69 to 1.1 per 100 catheterized patient-days.[3,8,17] The urinary tract of residents with chronic indwelling catheters is the most common source of bacteremia among long-term care facility residents. Bacteremia is reported to be 3 to 39 times more common in residents with chronic indwelling catheters.[4] At autopsy, there was histologic evidence of acute pyelonephritis in 38% of residents with a chronic indwelling catheter and only 5% without a catheter, whereas histologic evidence for chronic pyelonephritis correlated with the duration an indwelling catheter had been used.[4] Chronic indwelling catheter replacement is accompanied by bacteremia in about 4% of episodes, but has not been associated with negative clinical consequences. Other symptomatic presentations that may complicate long-term indwelling catheter use include urolithiasis, urethritis, periurethral abscesses, and epididymitis or prostatitis.

Reported rates of symptomatic urinary infection for patients managed with intermittent catheterization vary from 0.41 to 1.86 per 100 patient days. This variation reflects different definitions and methods used for case ascertainment among reported studies, and varying characteristics of the patient populations. The incidence of symptomatic infection in spinal cord–injured men managed with intermittent catheterization is 0.41 per 100 person-days, which is similar to men managed with condom catheters, at 0.36 per 100 person-days. This compares with 2.72 per 100 person-days for a similar population managed with chronic indwelling catheters.[4]

DIAGNOSIS
Clinical

Catheter-acquired urinary infection is usually asymptomatic. The most common symptomatic presentation for patients with indwelling catheters is fever without localizing genitourinary findings and no alternate source identified. The clinical diagnosis is usually a diagnosis of exclusion. Localizing signs and symptoms that are occasionally present include catheter obstruction, hematuria, and costovertebral angle or suprapubic pain or tenderness. However, the validity or reliability of any one or combination of these symptoms for diagnosis of urinary infection has not been critically evaluated. The usual localizing symptoms of lower urinary tract infection (frequency, urgency, dysuria, and stranguria) are useful for identification of infection only when symptom onset occurs after catheter removal. Other local suppurative presentations that occur primarily in patients with chronic indwelling catheters include urethritis, periurethral abscesses, epididymoorchitis, and prostatitis.

Consensus clinical criteria proposed for initiating antimicrobial therapy for presumed urinary infection in long-term care facility residents with an indwelling catheter include one or more of fever (>37.9°C or 1.5°C increase over baseline); new costovertebral angle tenderness; rigors; or new-onset delirium with no other apparent source.[18] This definition has been validated in a prospective, randomized trial and reported to be efficacious and safe for clinical management.[19] The National Healthcare Safety Network definitions for surveillance, rather than treatment, of catheter-acquired urinary infection in patients with short- or long-term catheters are summarized in **Box 1**.[2]

Neurologic impairment of individuals managed with intermittent catheterization may alter clinical presentations of symptomatic urinary infection. Lower tract irritative symptoms and costovertebral angle pain or tenderness may occur, but these patients also present with atypical symptoms, such as increased lower limb spasticity, incontinence, difficult catheterization because of obstruction or, in individuals with injury at a high cord level, autonomic dysreflexia.[4,20] These symptoms, however, have limited sensitivity or specificity for identifying bacteriuria.[21]

Box 1
Criteria for symptomatic urinary tract infection proposed by the National Healthcare Safety Network for catheter-acquired urinary infection

At least one of the following signs or symptoms with no other recognized cause: fever (>38°C), suprapubic tenderness, costovertebral angle pain or tenderness

or

For patient ≤1 year of age, one of fever (>38°C core), hypothermia (<36°C core), apnea bradycardia, dysuria, lethargy, or vomiting

and

Urine culture with ≥10^5 cfu/mL with no more than two species of microorganisms

or

Urine culture with ≥10^3 and <10^5 cfu/mL with no more than two species and positive urinalysis (one of positive dipstick for leukocyte esterase or nitrite; pyuria [≥10 wbc/mm³ or ≥3 wbc/hpf unspun urine]; microorganisms in Gram stain of unspun urine).

Data from Gould CV, Umscheid CA, Agarwal RK, et al. Guideline for prevention of catheter-associated urinary tract infections 2009. Available at: http://www.cdc.gov/hicpac/. Accessed January 14, 2011.

Urine Culture

A urine culture should be obtained before initiating antimicrobial therapy for any patient with suspected symptomatic urinary infection and an indwelling or intermittent catheter in situ. If a short-term indwelling catheter is in place, the specimen should be collected by puncture of the catheter sampling port or tubing. A urine specimen collected through a catheter with an established biofilm is contaminated by the biofilm and a greater number of organisms and higher quantitative counts are isolated compared with bladder urine.[22] Thus, when symptomatic infection is suspected and a catheter has been in place for a prolonged period, the catheter should be replaced by a new catheter and a urine specimen for culture collected immediately through the newly inserted catheter, before institution of antimicrobial therapy. This specimen samples bladder urine without biofilm contamination and is more relevant for antimicrobial management. The duration a catheter remains in situ before a recommendation for pretherapy catheter replacement is not clearly defined, but an interval of 2 weeks or longer is suggested.[4]

The quantitative criteria for diagnosis of asymptomatic bacteriuria in a patient with a short-term indwelling catheter is isolation of greater than or equal to 10^5 cfu/mL of one or more organisms from the urine specimen.[4] Initial lower bacterial counts of greater than or equal to 10^2 cfu/mL can increase to greater than or equal to 10^5 cfu/mL within 48 hours if the catheter remains in situ and antibiotics are not initiated.[23] These initial lower quantitative counts likely represent catheter biofilm colonization, and not bladder bacteriuria. For the patient with a chronic indwelling catheter, the quantitative count of greater than or equal to 10^5 cfu/mL of one or more organisms is also appropriate. When organisms are present at greater than or equal to 10^5 cfu/mL, concomitant organisms isolated from bladder urine at lower counts generally do not persist after catheter replacement and should be considered contaminants.[24] Biofilm contamination is not a consideration for specimens collected by in-and-out catheterization, intermittent catheterization, or a freshly inserted indwelling catheter in a patient without a prior catheter. For specimens collected with these catheters a lower quantitative count of greater than or equal to 10^2 cfu/mL is diagnostic for bacteriuria, although greater than or equal to 10^5 cfu/mL is isolated from most patients. When urine specimens collected by intermittent catheterization were compared with a reference suprapubic aspirate specimen, the optimal quantitative criteria to identify bacteriuria was greater than or equal to 10^2 cfu/mL, with a positive predictive value of 0.93 and negative predictive value of 0.96.[25]

Patients with a short-term indwelling catheter in situ who experience symptomatic infection usually have a quantitative count of greater than or equal to 10^5 cfu/mL isolated. Organisms growing in the residual pool of urine that persists in the bladder of patients with indwelling catheters have adequate time to achieve high concentrations. The frequency of isolation of organisms with a quantitative count less than 10^5 cfu/mL from patients presenting with symptomatic infection and a short-term indwelling catheter has not been reported. Lower quantitative counts may occur when patients are experiencing diuresis or receiving antimicrobial therapy, or may represent early biofilm contamination of the catheter. A prospective study of antimicrobial therapy for patients with a chronic indwelling catheter and presumed febrile urinary infection reported 23 (82%) of 28 patients had a quantitative count of greater than or equal to 10^5 cfu/mL in bladder urine collected after catheter replacement.[22] Organisms isolated at counts less than 10^5 cfu/mL after catheter replacement should be considered infecting organisms only if no other organisms are present at greater than or equal to 10^5 cfu/mL. When organisms are isolated only in lower quantitative counts from a patient with an indwelling chronic catheter, attribution of fever to a urinary tract source should be critically reassessed.

The National Institute on Disability and Rehabilitation recommends quantitative criteria of greater than or equal to 10^2 cfu/mL for diagnosis of urinary infection in symptomatic persons managed with intermittent catheterization.[20] However, when catheter specimens were compared with paired suprapubic aspirates, only one of five symptomatic patients had counts less than 10^5 cfu/mL.[25] In addition, in a prospective randomized clinical trial enrolling spinal cord–injured patients with symptomatic urinary infection that used a quantitative count of greater than or equal to 10^3 cfu/mL for identification of bacteriuria,[26] 37 (84%) of 44 subjects managed with intermittent catheterization had greater than or equal to 10^5 cfu/mL isolated (unpublished data). Thus, most patients practicing intermittent catheterization who present with symptomatic urinary infection have greater than or equal to 10^5 cfu/mL of organisms isolated.

Pyuria

Pyuria accompanies bacteriuria in virtually all individuals with catheter-acquired urinary infection.[4] For both short- and long-term indwelling catheters, the degree of pyuria is similar for asymptomatic or symptomatic infection. The indwelling catheter causes bladder irritation leading to inflammation and pyuria, even without bacteriuria. Thus, pyuria is ubiquitous in patients with indwelling catheters and has no diagnostic use for either identifying bacteriuria or differentiating symptomatic from asymptomatic infection.[4] Pyuria is also invariably associated with bacteriuria for patients maintained with intermittent catheterization, and does not distinguish between symptomatic or asymptomatic infection. The absence of pyuria, however, is useful to exclude bacteriuria in patients with catheters.[4]

TREATMENT
Asymptomatic Catheter-Acquired Urinary Tract Infection

Antibiotic treatment of asymptomatic catheter-acquired urinary tract infection is not recommended because morbidity, including symptomatic episodes, is not improved, whereas resistant organisms consistently emerge in subsequent infections.[27] A clinical trial in critical care unit patients reported that treatment of asymptomatic bacteriuria and catheter replacement compared with no intervention was not associated with any improved patient outcomes.[28] Treatment of asymptomatic candiduria in patients with indwelling urethral catheters also is not effective for eradicating funguria or improving clinical outcomes. In a placebo-controlled trial, 61% of fluconazole and 56% of placebo-treated patients cleared candiduria when assessed 2 weeks after treatment.[29] For patients with long-term indwelling catheters, antimicrobial treatment did not decrease the prevalence of asymptomatic bacteriuria or incidence of symptomatic urinary tract infection. However, subjects randomized to antimicrobial treatment had a significant increase in isolation of organisms resistant to the study antimicrobial in subsequent urine cultures.[4] Treatment of asymptomatic bacteriuria in persons using intermittent catheterization is also not recommended because of limited, if any, clinical benefit, and an increased frequency of resistant organisms isolated from subsequent infections.[27]

Symptomatic Catheter-Acquired Infection

Antimicrobial treatment of symptomatic infection must consider the known or suspected susceptibility of infecting organisms, clinical presentation, and patient tolerance and renal function. The antimicrobial selected should have substantial urinary excretion, achieving high urinary levels. Prior antimicrobial therapy received by the patient and local prevalence of antimicrobial resistance must also be considered. Patients who are severely ill with high fever, nausea or vomiting, or hemodynamic instability require initial empiric parenteral antimicrobial therapy. The antimicrobial regimen is reassessed after the urine culture results are available and the initial clinical response can be reviewed, usually at 48 to 72 hours of therapy. When patients present with symptoms that are mild or of questionable urinary origin, antimicrobial therapy should be delayed pending urine culture results so that specific antimicrobial therapy can be prescribed. There should be a prompt defervescence of fever after initiation of appropriate antimicrobial therapy for patients with adequate renal function and no complicating abnormalities, such as obstruction or abscesses. In a group of long-term care facility residents with presumed febrile urinary infection and catheter replacement before initiating antimicrobial therapy, 81% were afebrile by 72 hours.[22] Antimicrobial treatment for individuals who develop symptoms of urinary infection after catheter removal is similar to treatment for individuals without an indwelling catheter.

The optimal duration of antimicrobial therapy is an unresolved question. If the indwelling catheter remains in situ, a 7-day course is recommended to limit emergence of resistant organisms.[4] For the 68 patients with indwelling catheters enrolled in a comparative clinical trial of therapy for complicated urinary infection, levofloxacin, 750 mg for 5 days, was as effective for clinical outcomes as ciprofloxacin, 250 mg twice daily for 10 days, with microbiologic eradication of 78.9% for levofloxacin and 47.7% for ciprofloxacin.[30] This suggests, at least for some agents, a course as short as 5 days might be considered. However, subjects in this study were enrolled only if a susceptible organism was isolated, and it was not stated if the catheter was removed. For spinal cord–injured patients managed with intermittent catheterization, 3 days of ciprofloxacin was inferior to 14 days, with a significantly higher incidence of symptomatic relapse posttherapy in subjects treated for the shorter duration.[26] Thus, the optimal duration of antimicrobial therapy remains undefined, and likely differs for different patient populations with indwelling catheters.

PREVENTION
Guidelines

Recently published or updated evidence-based national and international guidelines systematically review recommendations for prevention of catheter-acquired urinary infection and highlight limitations of current evidence.[1,2,4,31] A concern for most studies that have evaluated preventive strategies is that outcomes are reported for asymptomatic bacteriuria rather than symptomatic urinary infection.[4] Prevention of catheter-acquired urinary infections in healthcare facilities is considered within the context of other quality assurance programs.[1,2] This requires written guidelines, adequate and appropriately trained staff, and monitoring of patient outcomes and staff compliance with recommended practices. Specific proposed outcome measures include frequency of catheter use, compliance with accepted indications for catheter use and removal, and occurrence of symptomatic infection and bacteremia.

Catheter Use

The preeminent strategy to limit catheter-acquired urinary tract infection is to minimize indwelling catheter use. An indwelling urinary catheter should be inserted only for approved indications (**Box 2**) and removed as soon as feasible.[1,2,4] From 20% to

---

Box 2
Appropriate indications for indwelling urethral catheter use identified by the Healthcare Infection Control Practices Advisory Committee

- Acute urinary retention or bladder outlet obstruction
- Accurate measurement of urine output in critically ill patients
- Selected perioperative use
  - Urologic or genitourinary surgery
  - Prolonged duration of surgery
  - Large-volume infusions or diuretics during surgery
  - Intraoperative monitoring of urine output
- Assist in healing open sacral or perineal wounds for incontinent patients
- Prolonged immobilization for spine or pelvic fractures
- Comfort for end-of-life care

Data from Gould CV, Umscheid CA, Agarwal RK, et al. Guideline for prevention of catheter-associated urinary tract infections 2009. Available at: http://www.cdc.gov/hicpac/. Accessed January 14, 2011.

50% of indwelling catheters inserted in acute-care facility patients do not meet appropriate indications, and 36% to 50% of catheter days are reported to be unjustified, because the catheter remains in situ beyond the minimum necessary time.[4] Several approaches are effective for limiting catheter use and duration. These include requiring a physician order for catheter insertion; physician or nurse daily reminders to reassess the need for a catheter; and nurse-initiated removal (stop orders) when specific predesignated criteria are met. Although these strategies are consistently effective in decreasing catheter use and bacteriuria,[32] the benefit for symptomatic infection is not established.[4,33]

Alternate methods of bladder emptying that avoid an indwelling urethral catheter, such as intermittent urinary catheterization and for men external condom catheters, should be considered whenever possible. There are no randomized comparative trials of intermittent catheterization compared with an indwelling catheter, but clinical experience and prospective and retrospective studies all support a decreased occurrence of symptomatic urinary infection with use of an intermittent catheter. Men using an external condom catheter have a lower frequency of symptomatic urinary infection than men with a chronic indwelling catheter.[2] A prospective, randomized trial of condom or indwelling catheter use for men in a Veterans Administration hospital reported a significantly improved composite outcome of bacteriuria, symptomatic infection, or death, and improved patient comfort, with the condom catheter.[34] The evidence to support a benefit with suprapubic catheterization is contradictory.[4] Decreased frequency of bacteriuria and increased patient comfort are reported for some studies. However, insertion of a suprapubic catheter requires a surgical procedure with attendant complications, and suprapubic catheter replacement requires specially trained personnel. Thus, current evidence is insufficient to recommend use of a suprapubic rather than indwelling urethral catheter for patients requiring either acute or chronic urinary catheterization.[4]

Catheter Care

Appropriate practices for catheter insertion and maintenance may delay acquisition of bacteriuria (**Box 3**).[1,2,4] These include aseptic insertion, maintenance of a closed

---

Box 3
Recommended practices for indwelling catheter insertion and maintenance

- Catheter insertion
  - Properly trained personnel
  - Hand hygiene
  - Smallest-bore catheter
  - Aseptic technique and sterile equipment
    - Sterile gloves, drapes, sponges, periurethral cleaning
    - Antiseptic lubricants not routine
- Catheter maintenance
  - Sterile, continuously closed drainage system
    - If breaks, replace catheter, collecting system, and connection
    - Consider using preconnected, sealed catheter-tubing junction
  - Maintain unobstructed urine flow from bladder to drainage bag
    - Avoid tube kinking
    - Keep bag below bladder
    - Empty bag regularly
    - Separate collecting containers for each patient
  - Standard precautions for catheter and collecting system manipulation

Data from Refs.[1,2,4]

---

drainage system, ensuring that the drainage tube and collection bag remain below the level of the bladder, and using a dedicated urine volume measuring container for each patient. Replacement of open by closed drainage for indwelling catheters in the 1960s revolutionized the frequency of infectious complications of catheter use. Subsequent studies have consistently reported more rapid acquisition of bacteriuria when there are breaks in the closed system.[4] Other recommended practices have more limited evidence to support efficacy in preventing infection. Several practices have evidence for lack of benefit and are no longer recommended, such as daily periurethral cleaning with an antiseptic or with green soap, or instillation of an antiseptic in the drainage bag. Shared urine volume measuring devices have been identified as a risk for transmission of bacteria among patients with indwelling catheters in hospital outbreaks of resistant bacteria.

Intermittent Catheter

A clean or sterile intermittent catheterization technique has similar outcomes for patients in the community or long-term care facilities. The clean technique is less costly, so is recommended for these settings. However, sterile technique for intermittent catheterization is still recommended for patients in acute-care facilities.[4] Intermittent catheters, if reused, should be cleaned and dried between uses. Prospective randomized comparative trials have not reported benefits of prophylactic antibiotics or of daily cranberry use to decrease symptomatic infection.[4] However, an intensive education program decreased bacteriuria and showed a trend to decreased episodes of symptomatic infection.[35] This program included provision of a consumer manual discussing aspects of urinary infection in spinal cord injury followed by a self-administered test together with physician and nurse review of individual patient catheter technique, hygiene, and urinary infection symptoms and telephone follow-up at 1 week.

Catheter Materials

Catheters are usually made of either latex or silicone, including silicone-coated latex catheters. There is no evidence for differential risks for bacteriuria or symptomatic infection for different catheter materials.[4] Silicone catheters may cause less urethral inflammation, resulting in decreased noninfectious complications, such as urethritis and stricture formation. The silicone catheter is also reported to be less subject to obstruction, but this is likely attributable to the larger lumen size of these catheters. Hydrogel-coated catheters have a low friction surface, which is alleged to decrease trauma to the urethra. There is in vitro evidence that a hydrogel coating modestly delays biofilm formation,[36] but clinical trials reported to date do not document any clinical benefits with use of these catheters. Clinical trials of hydrogel-coated catheters for subjects managed with intermittent catheterization have reported inconsistent results with respect to benefits.[2,4]

Antimicrobial-Coated Catheters

Another proposed approach to prevent catheter-associated urinary infection is to coat catheters with antibacterial materials. Early studies with a silver oxide–coated catheter reported no benefit for preventing bacteriuria, but silver alloy catheters were subsequently reported to decrease acquisition of bacteriuria, although symptomatic infection was not adequately evaluated.[37,38] A meta-analysis suggested the reported benefit of silver alloy catheters was only evident in early studies, and may have been confounded by the selection of the comparator catheter. A benefit for the silver alloy catheter was much less apparent when the control catheter was the same material as the test catheter (ie, silicone rather than latex).[39] A recent large, prospective, randomized study comparing a silver alloy hydrogel-coated silicone catheter with a silicone hydrogel-coated catheter reported no difference between the two catheters in acquisition of bacteriuria, incidence of symptomatic infection, or bacteremia.[14] In vitro studies of bacterial adherence also report no differences between a hydrogel catheter and silver alloy hydrogel catheter.[32] Thus, current evidence does not support a clinical benefit for use of silver alloy–coated indwelling catheters, and routine use of these catheters is not recommended.[1,2]

Nitrofurazone, an antimicrobial in the same class as nitrofurantoin, has also been used for catheter coating. Patients using these catheters had significantly decreased acquisition of bacteriuria for the initial 7 days after catheter insertion, but studies are not sufficiently powered to address the outcome of symptomatic infection.[4] In vitro studies report the nitrofurazone-coated catheter decreases E coli adherence and biofilm formation for up to 5 days, but the effect on Enterococcus spp. is for less than 48 hours.[40] Nitrofurazone, like nitrofurantoin, has poor efficacy for several bacterial species isolated from catheter-acquired urinary infection, such as K pneumoniae, P mirabilis, P aeruginosa, and P stuartii. Thus, these catheters have limited benefits for delaying bacteriuria and, to date, no evidence of clinical benefit.

Complex Catheter Systems

Modifications in catheter design, such as presealed junctions, iodine cartridges, bacterial filters, and backflow valves, have also been introduced as measures to decrease acquisition of infection.[4] Clinical trials of presealed catheter and tubing junctions report inconsistent results for efficacy in preventing bacteriuria.[4] Other catheter system modifications have not been shown to be effective for decreasing symptomatic catheter-acquired urinary tract infection or, in most cases, bacteriuria. For instance, a prospective, randomized trial in a critical care unit population compared a complex closed drainage system (preattached catheter, antireflux valve, drip chamber, and povidone–iodine releasing cartridge) with a simple two-chamber closed system and reported no difference in acquisition of bacteriuria by patients with the different catheters.[41]

Antimicrobial Therapy

Patients who receive antimicrobials have a decreased frequency of bacteriuria for the first 4 days of catheterization. Subsequently, infection acquisition is similar to that observed in patients not receiving an antimicrobial, and organisms acquired have increased antimicrobial resistance. Thus, prophylactic antimicrobial therapy is not recommended to prevent catheter-acquired bacteriuria.[4] Patients receiving antimicrobials for any indication at the time of catheter removal also have a lower prevalence of asymptomatic bacteriuria subsequently identified. The practice of antimicrobial therapy given at the time of catheter removal remains controversial. Comparative clinical trials report a decreased prevalence of bacteriuria at follow-up in some, but not all studies.[4] Women with catheter-acquired bacteriuria persisting 48 hours after removal of a short-term catheter had a decreased frequency of symptomatic infection in the subsequent 14 days with antimicrobial treatment compared with placebo.[4] However, further studies including a wider range of patient populations are necessary to define the benefits of treatment after catheter removal.

Other Interventions

Routine catheter changes are not recommended for patients with chronic indwelling catheters.[1,2,4] The catheter should only be changed with catheter obstruction, damage, or malfunction, or before treatment for symptomatic infection. The low risk of bacteremia observed when chronic indwelling catheters are changed has not been associated with any negative clinical outcomes. Thus, antimicrobial prophylaxis for catheter replacement is not recommended. Irrigation of an indwelling catheter is recommended only if obstruction from blood clots is anticipated. When irrigation is necessary, intermittent rather than continuous irrigation should be used, and the catheter and tubing junction disinfected before disconnection.[2]

SUMMARY

The urinary catheter is one of the most frequently used invasive medical devices. Patient exposure may be exceedingly short with a single catheterization or continue for years in individuals with chronic indwelling catheters. Biofilm formation along the catheter means that bacteriuria develops predictably if the indwelling catheter remains in situ. However, symptomatic infection is relatively uncommon for patients managed with short-term catheters. Prevention of infection includes limiting exposure by avoiding use of indwelling catheters and, when a catheter is used, removing it promptly when it is no longer indicated. Programs to limit catheter-acquired urinary infection should be implemented and monitored in all healthcare facilities where these devices are used. Appropriate management of symptomatic infection includes appreciating the increased likelihood of isolation of resistant organisms in these patients and the need to minimize antimicrobial exposure to limit further resistance emergence, and replacement of chronic indwelling catheters before institution of antimicrobial therapy.

The ultimate resolution of this clinical problem requires technologic advances including the development of biofilm-resistant catheter materials.

REFERENCES

1. Lo E, Nicolle L, Classen D, et al. Strategies to prevent catheter-associated urinary tract infections in acute care hospitals. Infect Control Hosp Epidemiol 2008;29: S41–50.
2. Gould CV, Umscheid CA, Agarwal RK, et al. Guideline for prevention of catheter-associated urinary tract infections 2009. Available at: http://www.cdc.gov/hicpac/. Accessed January 14, 2011.
3. Smith PW, Bennett G, Bradley S, et al. SHEA/APIC Guideline: infection prevention and control in the long term care facility. Infect Control Hosp Epidemiol 2008;29: 785–814.
4. Hooton TM, Bradley SE, Cardenas DD, et al. Diagnosis, prevention, and treatment of catheter-associated urinary tract infection in adults: 2009 international practice guidelines from the Infectious Diseases Society of America. Clin Infect Dis 2010;50:625–63.
5. Jacobson SM, Stickler DJ, Mobley HLT, et al. Complicated catheter-associated urinary tract infections due to *Escherichia coli* and *Proteus mirabilis*. Clin Microbiol Rev 2008;21:26–59.
6. Saint S, Chenowith CE. Biofilms and catheter-associated urinary tract infections. Infect Dis Clin North Am 2003;17:411–32.
7. Stickler DJ, Feneley RC. The encrustation and blockage of long-term indwelling bladder catheters: a way forward in prevention and control. Spinal Cord 2010; 48:784–90.
8. Warren JW, Damron D, Tenney JH, et al. Fever, bacteremia and death as complications of bacteriuria in women with long term urethral catheters. J Infect Dis 1987;155:1151–8.
9. Ouslander JG, Greengold B, Chen S. Complications of chronic indwelling urinary catheters among male nursing home patients. A prospective study. J Urol 1987; 138:1191–5.
10. Johnson JR, Roberts PL, Stamm WE. *P fimbriae* and other virulence factors in *Escherichia coli* urosepsis: association with patients' characteristics. J Infect Dis 1987;156:225–9.
11. Watts RE, Hancock V, Ong CL, et al. *Escherichia coli* isolates causing asymptomatic bacteriuria in catheterized and noncatheterized individuals possess similar virulence properties. J Clin Microbiol 2010;48:2449–58.
12. Bakke A, Vollset SE. Risk factors for bacteriuria and clinical urinary tract infection in patients treated with clean intermittent catheterization. J Urol 1993;149: 527–31.
13. Tambyah PA, Maki DG. Catheter-associated urinary tract infection is rarely symptomatic: a prospective study of 1,497 catheterized patients. Arch Intern Med 2000;160:678–82.
14. Srinivasan A, Karchmer T, Richards A, et al. A prospective trial of a novel, silicone-based, silver-coated Foley catheter for the prevention of nosocomial urinary tract infection. Infect Control Hosp Epidemiol 2006;27:38–43.
15. Warren JW, Tenney JH, Hoopes HM, et al. A prospective microbiologic study of bacteriuria in patients with chronic indwelling urethral catheters. J Infect Dis 1982;146:719–23.
16. Nicolle LE. Catheter-related urinary tract infection. Drugs Aging 2005;22:627–39.

17. Orr PH, Nicolle LE, Duckworth H, et al. Febrile urinary infection in the institution-alized elderly. Am J Med 1996;100:71–7.
18. Loeb M, Bentley DW, Bradley S, et al. Development of minimum criteria for the initiation of antibiotics in residents of long term care facilities: results of a consensus conference. Infect Control Hosp Epidemiol 2001;22:120–4.
19. Loeb M, Brazil K, Lohfeld L, et al. Effect of a multifaceted intervention on number of antimicrobial prescriptions for suspected urinary tract infections in residents of nursing homes: cluster randomized controlled trial. BMJ 2005; 331:669.
20. National Institute on Disability and Rehabilitation Research Consensus State-ment. The prevention and management of urinary tract infections among people with spinal cord injuries. J Am Paraplegia Soc 1992;15:194–204.
21. Massa LM, Hoffman JM, Cardenas DD. Validity accuracy, and predictive value of urinary tract infection signs and symptoms in individuals with spinal cord injury on intermittent catheterization. J Spinal Cord Med 2009;32:568–73.
22. Raz R, Schiller D, Nicolle LE. Chronic indwelling catheter replacement before antimicrobial therapy for symptomatic urinary tract infection. J Urol 2000;164: 1254–8.
23. Stark RP, Maki DG. Bacteriuria in the catheterized patient. What quantitative level of bacteriuria is relevant? N Engl J Med 1984;311:560–4.
24. Tenney JH, Warren JW. Bacteriuria in women with long-term catheters: paired comparison of indwelling and replacement catheters. J Infect Dis 1988;157: 199–202.
25. Gribble MJ, McCallum NM, Schechter MT. Evaluation of diagnostic criteria for bacteriuria in acutely spinal cord injured patients undergoing intermittent cathe-terization. Diagn Microbiol Infect Dis 1988;9:197–206.
26. Dow G, Rao P, Harding G, et al. A prospective, randomized trial of 3 or 14 days of ciprofloxacin treatment for acute urinary tract infections in patients with spinal cord injury. Clin Infect Dis 2004;39:658–64.
27. Nicolle LE, Bradley S, Colgan R, et al. IDSA guideline for the diagnosis and treat-ment of asymptomatic bacteriuria in adults. Clin Infect Dis 2005;40:643–54.
28. Leone M, Perrin AS, Granier I, et al. A randomized trial of catheter change and short course antibiotics for asymptomatic bacteriuria in catheterized ICU patients. Intensive Care Med 2007;33:726–9.
29. Sobel JD, Kauffman CA, McKinsey D, et al. Candiduria: a randomized, double blind study of treatment with fluconazole or placebo. Clin Infect Dis 2000;30:19–24.
30. Peterson J, Kaul S, Khashab M, et al. A double-blind, randomized comparison of levofloxacin 750 mg once-daily for five days with ciprofloxacin 400/500 mg twice daily for 10 days for the treatment of complicated urinary tract infections and acute pyelonephritis. Urology 2008;71:17–22.
31. Pratt RJ, Pellowe CM, Wilson JA, et al. EPIC 2: National evidence-based guide-lines for preventing healthcare-associated infections in NHS hospitals in England. J Hosp Infect 2007;65(Suppl 1):S1–64.
32. Meddings J, Rogers MA, Macy M, et al. Systemic review and meta-analysis: reminder systems to reduce catheter-associated urinary tract infections and urinary catheter use in hospitalized patients. Clin Infect Dis 2010;51:550–60.
33. Loeb M, Hunt D, O'Halloran K, et al. Stop orders to reduce inappropriate urinary catheterization in hospitalized patients: a randomized controlled trial. J Gen Intern Med 2008;23:16–20.
34. Saint S, Kaufman SR, Rogers MA, et al. Condom vs indwelling urinary catheters: a randomized trial. J Am Geriatr Soc 2006;54:1055–61.

35. Cardenas DD, Hoffman JM, Kelly E, et al. Impact of a urinary tract infection educational program in persons with spinal cord injury. J Spinal Cord Med 2004;27:47–54.
36. Desai DG, Liao KS, Cervallos ME, et al. Silver or nitrofurazone impregnation of urinary catheters has a minimal effect on uropathogen adherence. J Urol 2010; 184:2565–71.
37. Johnson JR, Kuskowski MA, Wilt TJ. Systematic review: antimicrobial urinary catheters to prevent catheter-associated urinary tract infection in hospitalized patients. Ann Intern Med 2006;144:116–27.
38. Niel-Weisse BS, Arend SM, van den Brock PJ. Is there evidence for recommending silver-coated urinary catheters in guidelines? J Hosp Infect 2002;52:81–7.
39. Crnech CJ, Drinka PJ. Does the composition of urinary catheter influence clinical outcomes and the results of research studies? Infect Control Hosp Epidemiol 2007;28:102–3.
40. Johnson JR, Johnston BD, Kuskowski MA, et al. In vitro activity of available antimicrobial coated Foley catheters against *Escherichia coli* including strains resistant to extended-spectrum cephalosporins. J Urol 2010;184:2572–7.
41. Leone M, Garnier F, Antonini F, et al. Comparison of effectiveness of two urinary drainage systems in intensive care unit: a prospective randomized clinical trial. Intensive Care Med 2003;29:551–4.

Management and Prevention of Prosthetic Joint Infection

Emily K. Shuman, MD[a], Andrew Urquhart, MD[b],
Preeti N. Malani, MD, MSJ[c],*

KEYWORDS

- Surgical site infections • Antimicrobials • Aging

Each year hundreds of thousands of patients undergo prosthetic replacement of knees, hips, shoulders, elbows, and even ankles, making total joint arthroplasty (TJA) one of the most common surgical procedures worldwide. Prosthetic joint infection (PJI) remains a feared and potentially devastating complication of TJA. Because joint replacement surgeries comprise mostly total knee arthroplasty (TKA) and total hip arthroplasty (THA), PJI related to these 2 procedures is the focus of this review.

PJIs can result in significant morbidity and functional impairment. Patients who develop PJI typically require extended hospitalization, additional surgical procedures, and long courses of parenteral antimicrobials. Although the overall rate of PJI after TJA is low (0.6%–1.6% for TKA and 0.7%–2.4% for THA),[1] the absolute number is significant (and growing), given the amount of procedures. PJIs also represent a significant economic burden, with associated health care costs topping $280 million annually in the United States.[2]

PATHOGENESIS AND RISK FACTORS

PJIs are generally classified according to the timing after surgery: early-onset infection occurs within 3 months after arthroplasty, delayed-onset infection within 3 to 24 months, and late-onset infection after 24 months[3]; the distribution of patients presenting within each category is approximately equal. As with other surgical site infections (SSIs),

The authors have nothing to disclose. There was no outside support for this work.
[a] Division of Infectious Diseases and Geriatric Medicine, University of Michigan, Ann Arbor, MI, USA
[b] Department of Orthopedic Surgery, University of Michigan, Ann Arbor, MI, USA
[c] Department of Internal Medicine, Divisions of Infectious Diseases and Geriatric Medicine, University of Michigan and Ann Arbor Veterans Affairs Ann Arbor Healthcare System, Geriatric Research Education and Clinical Center, 2215 Fuller Road, 111-I, 8th Floor, Ann Arbor, MI 48105, USA
* Corresponding author.
E-mail address: pmalani@umich.edu

PJIs occur most commonly because of contamination of the surgical wound with locally introduced microorganisms.[4] Therefore, anything that delays wound healing increases the risk of PJI. Although the risk of infection is primarily related to microbial inoculum, other factors such as the virulence of the microorganisms, patient-related factors, and procedure-related factors help determine susceptibility to infection. Prosthetic joints can also become infected via secondary spread related to bloodstream infections; the most common sources are skin and soft tissue, dental sources, and the urinary tract.[5]

Risk factors for PJI can be broadly divided into patient-related and procedure-related risks. Important patient-related risk factors for PJI include a history of prior PJI as well as a concurrent infection at the time of surgery (eg, another SSI or wound infection, urinary tract infection, pressure ulcers).[3,6,7] Several comorbid conditions are associated with increased PJI risk, including diabetes mellitus, rheumatoid arthritis, psoriasis, immunocompromised state, malignancy, corticosteroid use, and obesity.[3,8,9] Although advanced age in itself does not seem to increase the risk of PJI,[3,6] dependence in activities of daily living has been associated with higher rates of SSI.[10,11]

Procedure-related risk factors include revision arthroplasty, extended operative duration (>2.5 hours), higher number of operating room personnel, postoperative bleeding or hematoma formation, and need for postoperative blood transfusion.[9,12,13] Simultaneous bilateral arthroplasty was traditionally believed to be a risk factor for PJI, but more recent studies suggest this is not the case.[14,15] However, many surgeons prefer to avoid this approach, given the potential increased need for blood transfusion, which does boost the risk of PJI. Bloodstream infection is another important risk factor because bioprosthetic material is highly susceptible to secondary infection from a hematogenous source.[3] In one prospective series, the incidence of PJI was 34% after *Staphylococcus aureus* bacteremia.[16] Once a prosthesis is seeded with microorganisms, either at the time of surgery or because of secondary spread, a biofilm typically forms, which cannot be eradicated using antimicrobials.[17]

MICROBIOLOGY

Almost any microorganism can be associated with PJI, but staphylococci (coagulase-negative staphylococci and *S aureus*) are the principal causative agents, accounting for more than half of all PJIs.[3,9] Other gram-positive and gram-negative bacilli each represent about 20% to 25% of infections, and anaerobes, including *Propionibacterium acnes*, account for another 10%. Polymicrobial infection is reported in 10% to 20% of PJIs. In a retrospective series of polymicrobial PJIs, the most frequently identified organisms included methicillin-resistant *S aureus* (MRSA) and anaerobes.[18] Approximately 10% of infections are culture negative. Although uncommon (approximately 1%), PJI associated with fungi and mycobacteria is described; increasing use of tumor necrosis factor α blockers among patients with joint disease may eventually increase the incidence of these and other unusual pathogens.

More virulent microorganisms, such as *S aureus* and gram-negative bacilli, are more likely to result in clinically apparent infection within 3 months after surgery (early-onset PJI), whereas less virulent microorganisms, such as coagulase-negative staphylococci and *P acnes*, are more likely to be associated with delayed-onset or late-onset infection.[9] Infection resulting from hematogenous seeding of prosthetic joints with a more virulent microorganism (specifically *S aureus*) can, however, occur at any time.

CLINICAL PRESENTATION AND DIAGNOSIS

Clinical manifestations of PJI are determined by several factors, including host characteristics, the route of infection, and associated microorganisms. The presentation can vary, ranging from a chronic indolent course characterized only by progressive joint pain to a fulminant septic arthritis; however, diagnosis is not always clear-cut because there are many noninfectious causes of prosthesis failure.

Patients with early-onset infection are more likely to have classic signs of inflammation and infection, including fever, erythema overlying the implant site, joint effusion, and/or wound drainage.[3,9] Patients with delayed-onset or late-onset infection generally have a more prolonged presentation with chronic joint pain, often with no typical signs of infection.[3,9] However, late-onset infection due to hematogenous seeding of the prosthesis can present with a more acute situation.[5] Typically, infection with more virulent microorganisms tends to produce more pronounced findings.[3] In contrast, less virulent organisms can simply present with progressive joint pain or loosening of the prosthesis in a manner that is indistinguishable from aseptic and mechanical complications.[3] Fever tends to be an unreliable indictor of PJI.

Although a simple gold standard to confirm PJI is lacking, diagnostic criteria have been proposed. The presence of 1 or more of the following criteria is believed to be adequate for PJI diagnosis: acute inflammation on histopathologic examination of periprosthetic tissue, sinus tract communicating with the prosthesis, gross purulence in the joint space, or growth of the same microorganism from 2 or more cultures of joint aspirates or periprosthetic tissue.[9]

In the absence of obvious physical examination signs and symptoms, further studies are required. Aspiration of joint synovial fluid is typically the most useful test for diagnosis of PJI, and there are established criteria for diagnosing PJI using this method.[9] Trampuz and colleagues[19] reported excellent results using arthrocentesis to diagnose prosthetic knee infection among patients without inflammatory joint disease using a cutoff value of white blood cell (WBC) count greater than 1700 cells/μL or a WBC differential greater than 65% polymorphonuclear leukocytes in the synovial fluid.

Laboratory markers, including WBC count, WBC differential, erythrocyte sedimentation rate (ESR), and C-reactive protein (CRP) level, are often elevated in those with PJI, but these numbers are neither specific nor sensitive and may be elevated because of other inflammatory conditions or, conversely, may be normal (especially among patients with delayed-onset or late-onset PJI).[9,20] Reported sensitivities and specificities of ESR range from 62% to 83% and 55% to 85%, respectively, and are only slightly better for CRP (60%–96% and 63%–92%, respectively).[9]

Imaging has an adjunctive role in PJI diagnosis, although most modalities have poor sensitivity and specificity. Patients with delayed-onset PJI may have evidence of loosening of the prosthesis or periosteal new bone formation on plain radiography, but these findings are again neither specific nor sensitive.[9] The use of computerized tomography and magnetic resonance imaging is limited by imaging artifacts related to the implant. Combined indium 111–labeled WBC and technetium 99m–labeled sulfur colloid scintigraphy has been reported to have a sensitivity of 80% to 86% and a specificity of 94% to 100%.[21,22] Positron emission tomography (PET) with fludeoxyglucose F 18 has been studied as a possible diagnostic modality, although its clinical utility remains undefined.[9,23–27]

If the diagnosis cannot be made preoperatively, the best approach is to obtain intraoperative periprosthetic tissue cultures to help establish the presence of PJI and to guide subsequent antimicrobial therapy. Because preceding antimicrobial therapy reduces the yield from both synovial fluid and operative cultures, antimicrobials should be stopped several days before revision arthroplasty to optimize yield.[3] The reported sensitivities of periprosthetic cultures vary from 53% to more than 90%.[3,6,28] Most experts recommend taking 3 or more samples from periprosthetic tissue with the most pronounced inflammation.[6,28] Atkins and colleagues[28] predicted a 94.8%

chance of true PJI if 3 or more cultures yielded the same organism for a patient who had 3 to 6 samples taken. The significance of a single positive culture is often unclear, but the growth of a virulent organism (S aureus), the presence of periprosthetic or synovial fluid purulence, the presence of a communicating sinus tract, as well as short time to culture positivity are all predictive of real infection.[3,29] A positive Gram stain also is highly suggestive of infection, although sensitivity is very poor.[30]

Molecular diagnostic techniques, although promising, remain largely investigational. The polymerase chain reaction may play a role in identification of difficult-to-culture or fastidious organisms or in patients administered antimicrobial treatment before surgery, although this is not being done routinely at most centers.[31] There is emerging evidence that sonication of the implant after removal can improve the yield of cultures by releasing organisms contained within the biofilm; however, this process is not yet widely available.[32]

TREATMENT

The ultimate goal of PJI treatment is to achieve a functional and pain-free joint; the approach requires a combination of medical and surgical therapies. Although treatment with antimicrobials alone is generally inadequate, patient preferences and the potential morbidity of further surgical intervention must be carefully considered. Although the most predictably effective approach involves removal of all foreign materials, patients who are unable or unwilling to undergo additional surgery can sometimes be managed with long-term suppressive antimicrobials if the intent is symptom management and not microbiological cure. Prosthesis stability is a key consideration, and, as a general rule, an unstable implant requires replacement. Otherwise, patient preference, the patient's suitability for additional surgery, duration of symptoms, microbiological test results, and soft tissue integrity are all-important factors.[3,6]

For patients who are candidates for additional surgery, there are several possible approaches (**Table 1**). The most conservative surgical approach is debridement with retention of device (DRD). Although DRD may include exchange of polymer components, the anchored portions of the prosthesis remain in place. Patients who have early-onset infection or acute onset of hematogenously acquired infection may undergo DRD followed by a prolonged course of antimicrobial therapy.[9] DRD is appropriate for patients who have had short duration of symptoms ($\leq$2–3 weeks) and have intact overlying soft tissue.[3,6,33–37] This approach is not appropriate for patients with unstable prostheses, sinus tract or abscess formation, or infection associated with difficult-to-treat organisms, including multidrug-resistant organisms. Treatment success and suppression of infection can be achieved in approximately 80% of appropriately selected cases.[3,34–37] By contrast, S aureus–associated PJI treated with DRD results in a very high 2-year failure rate, even among properly selected patients.[38] There is a growing consensus among orthopedic surgeons that DRD may not be a preferred approach for management of PJI compared with other surgical approaches.

For patients with delayed-onset infection, removal of the prosthesis is typically required. If a patient is not expected to gain significant function from replacement of the prosthesis, the prosthesis may simply be removed and may not be replaced. However, for most patients, the preferred approach is a staged replacement of the entire device, either as a single-stage exchange (SSE), whereby the whole implant (metallic prosthesis, cement, and accompanying biofilm) is replaced in a single procedure, or, more commonly, as a 2-stage exchange (TSE).[9] In TSE, the prosthesis is

Table 1
Surgical approaches for management of PJI

Surgical Approach	Indications	Contraindications
Debridement with retention of device	Stable prosthesis Good soft tissue integrity Early-onset infection (<1 mo after initial surgery) Short duration of symptoms before presentation (<10 d) Infection with less virulent microorganism	Unstable prosthesis Presence of sinus tract Extended duration of symptoms Infection with virulent microorganism
Single-stage exchange	Good soft tissue integrity Longer duration of symptoms (≥3 wk) Infection with less virulent microorganism	Poor quality of soft tissue or bony stock Presence of sinus tract Infection with virulent microorganism
Two-stage exchange	Extended course of infection before debridement Presence of sinus tract Infection with virulent microorganism	Poor quality of soft tissue or bony stock
Arthrodesis	Recurrent infection despite revision arthroplasty Poor bony stock or soft tissue Inability to tolerate further revision arthroplasty Infection with antimicrobial-resistant organisms	—
Amputation	Inability to tolerate further revision arthroplasty Poor bony stock or soft tissue, precluding other surgical options Failure of the treatment options mentioned earlier Infection with antimicrobial-resistant organisms	—

Data from Refs.[3,6,9,30–37]

removed and replaced temporarily with a polymethyl methacrylate spacer, often impregnated with antimicrobials. After 2 to 8 weeks, a new prosthesis is implanted. In addition to the surgical management, patients receive extended courses of antimicrobials.

For individuals with PJI associated with more virulent organisms (ie, *S aureus,* gram-negative organisms, fungi), compromised soft tissue, or prolonged symptoms (>3 weeks), TSE provides superior outcomes compared with more conservative approaches and can result in microbiological cure in 87% to 100% of cases.[6,39,40] The disadvantages of TSE include an increased number of surgical procedures and prolonged periods of immobility. SSE may be appropriate for patients who have had prolonged symptoms but otherwise have intact soft tissue and less virulent organisms. The success rate for SSE has been reported to be more than 75% in selected patients.[3,6,37] In cases in which infection cannot be controlled despite aggressive medical and surgical therapy, arthrodesis (fusion) and occasionally even amputation can be considered.

Although recommendations regarding optimal antimicrobial therapy vary, treatment typically consists of approximately 6 weeks of high-dose therapy (parenteral or parenteral equivalent) after surgery. Some clinicians favor follow-up courses of long-term oral therapy as suppressive or consolidation therapy if the device is retained. In all cases, the choice of antimicrobial agents should be based on cultures obtained from synovial fluid, periprosthetic tissue, or sonication of the removed prosthesis. Clinicians should consider issues such as tissue penetration, tolerability, and bacteri-cidal activity when selecting a treatment regimen.

The long-term use of oral antimicrobials, although widely applied as suppressive therapy for retained implants, remains controversial. No large controlled trials have established whether such therapy prevents or delays treatment failure.[3,34–36,41] Long-term suppressive therapy may be appropriate in individuals with well-fixed pros-theses infected with a relatively indolent organism or in patients who cannot tolerate or do not wish further surgical intervention.[35,41] In these cases, it is essential that the infecting organism be susceptible to an oral agent that can be well tolerated over long periods because the rate of adverse drug reactions is approximately 8% to 22% (even in the best of scenarios).[6] The ideal length of suppressive therapy remains unclear. Some have advocated lifelong antimicrobials, whereas others define the length of therapy at 3 months for THA infection and 6 months for TKA infection.[42–48] Decisions regarding the choice of suppressive agent and the length of therapy are generally based on clinician and patient preference, treatment failure, and adverse drug events.

PREVENTION

The general principles of SSI prevention apply to decreasing the risk of PJI.[46] Procedure-related prevention focuses on reducing microbial inoculum and preventing contamination of the surgical site. Specific strategies include preparation of the surgical site with an appropriate antiseptic agent, hand scrubbing and use of appro-priate attire by surgical staff, sterilization and disinfection of equipment, minimizing traffic in the operating room, and use of appropriate ventilation systems.[49] Other prevention strategies address modifiable patient-related factors such as tight periop-erative blood glucose control for patients with diabetes and minimizing use of immu-nosuppressive medications. Appropriate use of perioperative systemic antimicrobial prophylaxis is another key to reducing the microbial inoculum that may be introduced into the surgical site. The specifics of surgical infection prophylaxis for prosthetic joint surgery have been reviewed in detail elsewhere.[50] The timing of administration of prophylactic antimicrobials is critical with the goal of achieving adequate serum and tissue minimum inhibitory concentrations against microorganisms expected to be encountered during surgery.

Colonization with S aureus or MRSA is known to be a risk factor for development of SSI.[51] The goal of preoperative screening for S aureus or MRSA carriage is to identify patients colonized with these organisms and to eradicate carriage through decoloni-zation. Decolonization is typically attempted using intranasal mupirocin, bathing with chlorhexidine-containing products, or both. Several randomized trials have tried to determine whether preoperative screening and decolonization for S aureus or MRSA carriage have an impact on SSI risk.[52–54] Recent SSI prevention guidelines suggest that preoperative screening and decolonization programs may be considered for patients undergoing orthopedic procedures, but this is not a conclusive recom-mendation. At present, this remains an unresolved issue.[49]

Use of antimicrobial-containing materials for prevention and treatment of ortho-pedic implant infection has become increasingly common. Antimicrobial-loaded bone cements have been used for more than 3 decades for treatment and prophylaxis but have only been approved by the US Food and Drug Administration within the past decade.[55] Cements can be hand mixed using a variety of antimicrobial agents or can be obtained premixed, typically containing tobramycin or gentamicin. Low concentrations of antimicrobials (eg, 600 mg of tobramycin per package of cement) are typically used for prophylaxis, whereas higher concentrations (eg, 1.2–3.6 g of tobramycin per package of cement) are used for treatment of PJI for patients undergoing TSE. One randomized study examined the efficacy of cefuroxime-impregnated bone cement (vs standard cement) on PJI prevention after TKA and found that patients receiving antimicrobial cement had lower rates of early-onset and delayed-onset PJI.[56] Two additional randomized trials found no difference in infection rates when comparing antimicrobial-loaded bone cements with standard systemic antimicrobial prophylaxis.[57,58] Two retrospective studies using large population registries from Europe demonstrated potential benefit with antimicrobial-loaded bone cements for prevention of PJI.[59,60]

Questions remain about what constitutes appropriate use of antimicrobial-loaded bone cements for prophylaxis. Some investigators advocate routine use of this practice, whereas others take a more selective approach, recommending use of antimicrobial-loaded bone cements for high-risk patients or in the setting of revision arthroplasty.[55,61] Potential concerns surrounding routine use of antimicrobial-loaded cement include development of antimicrobial resistance, compromise of the cement's mechanical properties, allergic reactions, and increased cost.

Another area of debate is the use of antimicrobial prophylaxis with dental procedures to prevent PJI. In 2003, the American Academy of Orthopedic Surgery (AAOS), American Dental Society, and Infectious Diseases Society of America published a guideline stating that prophylaxis for dental procedures should not be used routinely but could be considered in very-high-risk patients.[62] However, in 2009, the AAOS published an information statement recommending that prophylaxis be used routinely after TJA in all patients.[63] Despite the AAOS information statement, evidence to support routine antimicrobial prophylaxis is lacking.[64] Other professional societies continue to adhere to the 2003 guideline and do not recommend routine prophylaxis for patients who have undergone TJA undergoing dental procedures.

SUMMARY

PJI can result in significant morbidity, especially in older adults with underlying functional impairment. Diagnosis of PJI is challenging and often cannot be firmly established until the prosthesis is removed. Management of PJI often requires removal of the prosthesis combined with an extended duration of antimicrobial treatment. Prevention of PJI requires a multifaceted approach, including perioperative antimicrobial prophylaxis. Related prevention measures that remain controversial include preoperative screening and decolonization, antimicrobial-loaded bone cements, and postoperative antimicrobial prophylaxis with dental procedures. As the number of TJAs performed continues to increase, additional research is needed to determine optimal approaches for the treatment and prevention of PJI.

REFERENCES

1. Edwards JR, Peterson KD, Mu Y, et al. National Healthcare Safety Network (NHSN) report: data summary for 2006 through 2008, issued December 2009. Am J Infect Control 2009;37:783–805.

2. Hellmann M, Mehta SD, Bishai DM, et al. The estimated magnitude and direct hospital costs of prosthetic joint infections in the United States, 1997 to 2004. J Arthroplasty 2010;25:766–71.

3. Zimmerli W, Trampuz A, Ochsner PE. Prosthetic-joint infections. N Engl J Med 2004;351:1645–54.

4. Dellinger EP, Ehrenkranz NJ, Jarvis WR. Surgical site infections. In: Jarvis WR, editor. Bennett and Brachman's hospital infections. 5th edition. Philadelphia: Lippincott, Williams & Wilkins; 2007. p. 583–98.

5. Maderazo EG, Judson S, Pasternak H. Late infections of total joint prostheses. A review and recommendations for prevention. Clin Orthop Relat Res 1988;(229): 131–42.

6. Sia IG, Berbari EF, Karchmer AW. Prosthetic joint infections. Infect Dis Clin N Am 2005;19:885–914.

7. Tsukayama DT, Estrada R, Gustilo RB. Infection after total hip arthroplasty. A study of the treatment of one hundred and six infections. J Bone Joint Surg Am 1996;78:512–23.

8. Berbari EF, Hanssen AD, Duffy MC, et al. Risk factors for prosthetic joint infection: case-control study. Clin Infect Dis 1998;27:1247–54.

9. Del Pozo JL, Patel R. Clinical practice. Infection associated with prosthetic joints. N Engl J Med 2009;361:787–94.

10. Anderson DJ, Chen LF, Schmader KE, et al. Poor functional status as a risk factor for surgical site infection due to methicillin-resistant *Staphylococcus aureus*. Infect Control Hosp Epidemiol 2008;29:832–9.

11. Shuman EK, Malani PN. Preventing surgical site infections in older adults: the need for a new approach. Aging Health 2008;4:567–9.

12. Poss R, Thornhill TS, Ewald FC, et al. Factors influencing the incidence and outcome of infection following total joint arthroplasty. Clin Orthop Relat Res 1984;(182):117–26.

13. Parvizi J, Ghanem E, Joshi A, et al. Does "excessive" anticoagulation predispose to periprosthetic infection? J Arthroplasty 2007;22(6 Suppl 2):24–8.

14. Berend ME, Ritter MA, Harty LD, et al. Simultaneous bilateral versus unilateral total hip arthroplasty an outcomes analysis. J Arthroplasty 2005;20:421–6.

15. Ritter MA, Harty LD, Davis KE, et al. Simultaneous bilateral, staged bilateral, and unilateral total knee arthroplasty. A survival analysis. J Bone Joint Surg Am 2003; 85:1532–7.

16. Murdoch DR, Roberts SA, Fowler VG Jr, et al. Infection of orthopedic prostheses after *Staphylococcus aureus* bacteremia. Clin Infect Dis 2001;32:647–9.

17. del Pozo JL, Patel R. The challenge of treating biofilm-associated bacterial infections. Clin Pharmacol Ther 2007;82:204–9.

18. Marculescu CE, Cantey JR. Polymicrobial prosthetic joint infections: risk factors and outcome. Clin Orthop Relat Res 2008;466:1397–404.

19. Trampuz A, Hanssen AD, Osmon DR, et al. Synovial fluid leukocyte count and differential for the diagnosis of prosthetic knee infection. Am J Med 2004;117:556–62.

20. Bare J, MacDonald SJ, Bourne RB. Preoperative evaluations in revision total knee arthroplasty. Clin Orthop Relat Res 2006;446:40–4.

21. Palestro CJ, Swyer AJ, Kim CK, et al. Infected knee prosthesis: diagnosis with In-111 leukocyte, Tc-99m sulfur colloid, and Tc-99m MDP imaging. Radiology 1991; 179:645–8.

22. Teller RE, Christie MJ, Martin W, et al. Sequential indium-labeled leukocyte and bone scans to diagnose prosthetic joint infection. Clin Orthop Relat Res 2000;(373):241–7.

23. Delank KS, Schmidt M, Michael JW, et al. The implications of 18F-FDG PET for the diagnosis of endoprosthetic loosening and infection in hip and knee arthroplasty: results from a prospective, blinded study. BMC Musculoskelet Disord 2006;7:20.

24. Love C, Marwin SE, Tomas MB, et al. Diagnosing infection in the failed joint replacement: a comparison of coincidence detection 18F-FDG and 111In-labeled leukocyte/99mTc-sulfur colloid marrow imaging. J Nucl Med 2004;45: 1864–71.

25. Mumme T, Reinartz P, Alfer J, et al. Diagnostic values of positron emission tomography versus triple-phase bone scan in hip arthroplasty loosening. Arch Orthop Trauma Surg 2005;125:322–9.

26. Stumpe KD, Notzli HP, Zanetti M, et al. FDG PET for differentiation of infection and aseptic loosening in total hip replacements: comparison with conventional radiography and three-phase bone scintigraphy. Radiology 2004;231:333–41.

27. Stumpe KD, Romero J, Ziegler O, et al. The value of FDG-PET in patients with painful total knee arthroplasty. Eur J Nucl Med Mol Imaging 2006;33:1218–25.

28. Atkins BL, Athanasou N, Deeks JJ, et al. Prospective evaluation of criteria for microbiological diagnosis of prosthetic-joint infection at revision arthroplasty. The OSIRIS Collaborative Study Group. J Clin Microbiol 1998;36:2932–9.

29. Athanasou NA, Pandey R, de Steiger R, et al. Diagnosis of infection by frozen section during revision arthroplasty. J Bone Joint Surg Br 1995;77:28–33.

30. Chimento GF, Finger S, Barrack RL. Gram stain detection of infection during revision arthroplasty. J Bone Joint Surg Br 1996;78:838–9.

31. Tarkin IS, Dunman PM, Garvin KL. Improving the treatment of musculoskeletal infections with molecular diagnostics. Clin Orthop Relat Res 2005;(437):83–8.

32. Trampuz A, Piper KE, Jacobson MJ, et al. Sonication of removed hip and knee prostheses for diagnosis of infection. N Engl J Med 2007;357:654–63.

33. Burger RR, Basch T, Hopson CN. Implant salvage in infected total knee arthroplasty. Clin Orthop Relat Res 1991;(273):105–12.

34. Everts RJ, Chambers ST, Murdoch DR, et al. Successful antimicrobial therapy and implant retention for streptococcal infection of prosthetic joints. ANZ J Surg 2004;74:210–4.

35. Marculescu CE, Berbari EF, Hanssen AD, et al. Outcome of prosthetic joint infections treated with debridement and retention of components. Clin Infect Dis 2006; 42:471–8.

36. Meehan AM, Osmon DR, Duffy MC, et al. Outcome of penicillin-susceptible streptococcal prosthetic joint infection treated with debridement and retention of the prosthesis. Clin Infect Dis 2003;36:845–9.

37. Pavoni GL, Giannella M, Falcone M, et al. Conservative medical therapy of prosthetic joint infections: retrospective analysis of an 8-year experience. Clin Microbiol Infect 2004;10:831–7.

38. Brandt CM, Sistrunk WW, Duffy MC, et al. *Staphylococcus aureus* prosthetic joint infection treated with debridement and prosthesis retention. Clin Infect Dis 1997; 24:914–9.

39. Lentino JR. Prosthetic joint infections: bane of orthopedists, challenge for infectious disease specialists. Clin Infect Dis 2003;36:1157–61.

40. Lieberman JR, Callaway GH, Salvati EA, et al. Treatment of the infected total hip arthroplasty with a two-stage reimplantation protocol. Clin Orthop Relat Res 1994;(301):205–12.

41. Segreti J, Nelson JA, Trenholme GM. Prolonged suppressive antibiotic therapy for infected orthopedic prostheses. Clin Infect Dis 1998;27:711–3.

42. Trampuz A, Zimmerli W. Prosthetic joint infections: update in diagnosis and treatment. Swiss Med Wkly 2005;135:243–51.
43. Drancourt M, Stein A, Argenson JN, et al. Oral rifampin plus ofloxacin for treatment of *Staphylococcus*-infected orthopedic implants. Antimicrob Agents Chemother 1993;37:1214–8.
44. Konig DP, Schierholz JM, Munnich U, et al. Treatment of staphylococcal implant infection with rifampicin-ciprofloxacin in stable implants. Arch Orthop Trauma Surg 2001;121:297–9.
45. Zimmerli W, Widmer AF, Blatter M, et al. Role of rifampin for treatment of orthopedic implant-related staphylococcal infections: a randomized controlled trial. Foreign-Body Infection (FBI) Study Group. JAMA 1998;279:1537–41.
46. Chuard C, Herrmann M, Vaudaux P, et al. Successful therapy of experimental chronic foreign-body infection due to methicillin-resistant *Staphylococcus aureus* by antimicrobial combinations. Antimicrob Agents Chemother 1991;35:2611–6.
47. Lucet JC, Herrmann M, Rohner P, et al. Treatment of experimental foreign body infection caused by methicillin-resistant *Staphylococcus aureus*. Antimicrob Agents Chemother 1990;34:2312–7.
48. Brause BD. Infected total knee replacement: diagnostic, therapeutic, and prophylactic considerations. Orthop Clin N Am 1982;13:245–9.
49. Anderson DJ, Kaye KS, Classen D, et al. Strategies to prevent surgical site infections in acute care hospitals. Infect Control Hosp Epidemiol 2008;29(Suppl 1): S51–61.
50. Shuman EK, Malani PN. Prevention and management of prosthetic joint infection in older adults. Drugs Aging 2011;28:13–26.
51. Wenzel RP, Perl TM. The significance of nasal carriage of *Staphylococcus aureus* and the incidence of postoperative wound infection. J Hosp Infect 1995;31: 13–24.
52. Perl TM, Cullen JJ, Wenzel RP, et al. Intranasal mupirocin to prevent postoperative *Staphylococcus aureus* infections. N Engl J Med 2002;346:1871–7.
53. Harbarth S, Fankhauser C, Schrenzel J, et al. Universal screening for methicillin-resistant *Staphylococcus aureus* at hospital admission and nosocomial infection in surgical patients. JAMA 2008;299:1149–57.
54. Bode LG, Kluytmans JA, Wertheim HF, et al. Preventing surgical-site infections in nasal carriers of *Staphylococcus aureus*. N Engl J Med 2010;362:9–17.
55. Hanssen AD. Prophylactic use of antibiotic bone cement: an emerging standard–in opposition. J Arthroplasty 2004;19(4 Suppl 1):73–7.
56. Chiu FY, Chen CM, Lin CF, et al. Cefuroxime-impregnated cement in primary total knee arthroplasty: a prospective, randomized study of three hundred and forty knees. J Bone Joint Surg Am 2002;84:759–62.
57. McQueen MM, Hughes SP, May P, et al. Cefuroxime in total joint arthroplasty. Intravenous or in bone cement. J Arthroplasty 1990;5:169–72.
58. Josefsson G, Kolmert L. Prophylaxis with systematic antibiotics versus gentamicin bone cement in total hip arthroplasty. A ten-year survey of 1,688 hips. Clin Orthop Relat Res 1993;(292):210–4.
59. Espehaug B, Engesaeter LB, Vollset SE, et al. Antibiotic prophylaxis in total hip arthroplasty. Review of 10,905 primary cemented total hip replacements reported to the Norwegian arthroplasty register, 1987 to 1995. J Bone Joint Surg Br 1997; 79:590–5.
60. Malchau H, Herberts P, Ahnfelt L. Prognosis of total hip replacement in Sweden. Follow-up of 92,675 operations performed 1978–1990. Acta Orthop Scand 1993; 64:497–506.

61. Dunbar MJ. Antibiotic bone cements: their use in routine primary total joint arthroplasty is justified. Orthopedics 2009;32(9):pii. DOI:10.3928/01477447-20090728-20.
62. American Dental Association, American Academy of Orthopedic Surgeons. Antibiotic prophylaxis for dental patients with total joint replacements. J Am Dent Assoc 2003;137:895–9.
63. American Academy of Orthopaedic Surgeons. Information statement: antibiotic prophylaxis for bacteremia in patients with joint replacements. Available at: www.aaos.org/about/papers/advistmt/1033.asp. Accessed May 26, 2011.
64. Berbari EF, Osmon DR, Carr A, et al. Dental procedures as risk factors for prosthetic hip or knee infection: a hospital-based prospective case-control study. Clin Infect Dis 2010;50:8–16.

Vascular Graft Infections

Michael H. Young, MD[a],*, Gilbert R. Upchurch Jr, MD[b],
Preeti N. Malani, MD, MSJ[c]

KEYWORDS

- Vascular graft infection • Biofilms • Prosthetic graft
- Arterial graft

Prosthetic vascular grafts represent an important advance in the management of chronic conditions such as peripheral arterial occlusive disease and arterial aneurysms, and as arteriovenous (AV) access for chronic hemodialysis. The rate of vascular graft infection (VGI) varies, with the incidence ranging from less than 1% for abdominal aortic grafts, to 2.6% for lower extremity grafts, to approximately 6% for infrainguinal vascular grafts[1–3]; in fact, some series suggest the rate of infection may be increasing.[4] The rate of infection in prosthetic arteriovenous hemodialysis grafts (AVHGs) is approximately 3.5%.[5] The medical and economic costs of VGI are substantial, with costs of medical and surgical therapy for a single episode of VGI estimated at US$40,000.[6] The mortality related to VGI has been reported between 13% and 58%, and the amputation rate in survivors varies between 8% and 52%.[7–11] Similarly, estimates suggest that 20% to 36% of all deaths in hemodialysis patients are related to infectious complications.[5] This review highlights the epidemiology, pathogenesis, diagnosis, management, and prevention of VGIs.

PATHOGENESIS

Biofilms are a polymeric matrix produced by microorganisms as they adhere to surfaces, and play an essential role in VGI and other implant infections.[12,13] From a pathogenesis viewpoint, biofilms represent a unique stage of growth in which

There was no outside support for this work.
The authors have nothing to disclose.
[a] Division of Infectious Diseases, University of Kentucky School of Medicine, University of Kentucky, 800 Rose Street, MN-672, Lexington, KY 40536, USA
[b] Department of Surgery, University of Virginia, PO Box 800679, Charlottesville, VA 22908-0679, USA
[c] Department of Internal Medicine, Divisions of Infectious Diseases and Geriatric Medicine, University of Michigan and Ann Arbor Veterans Affairs Ann Arbor Healthcare System, Geriatric Research Education and Clinical Center, 2215 Fuller Road, 111-I, 8th Floor, Ann Arbor, MI 48105, USA
* Corresponding author.
E-mail address: myoun4@uky.edu

microorganisms are relatively resistant to host immune mechanisms. Biofilms can develop on living or inert tissue, though they preferentially occur on artificial materials or dead tissue.[12] In fact, the presence of a foreign body reduces the inoculum of *Staphylococcus aureus* needed to cause infection by a factor of 100,000.[14] Within the biofilms, microorganisms display phenotypic phase variation between an embedded, sessile form and a free-floating, planktonic state.[13] The sessile form is responsible for adhesion and biofilm formation, whereas the planktonic form is responsible for dissemination. Microorganisms in the sessile stage are comparatively phenotypically inert, but exhibit complex metabolic changes and organized behavior much different to what would be expected normally.[12]

Prosthetic grafts can become colonized via direct, contiguous invasion or via hematogenous seeding. The likelihood of an implant becoming colonized or infected will vary depending on type and structure of the material involved (eg, braided sutures are more likely to become infected than monofilament and woven Dacron is more susceptible than polytetrafluoroethylene)[1] as well as the microbes involved, which in large part depend on anatomic site.[2]

Sessile microorganisms within biofilms are resistant to killing by both host immunity and antimicrobial agents. The mechanisms of this resistance are not fully understood, but appear to be due to multiple factors. Artificial implants stimulate a chronic, low-grade inflammatory response that results in an immunoincompetent zone that impairs phagocyte bactericidal capacity, but also leads to peri-implant tissue damage and increases the likelihood of implant failure and infection.[13] Microorganisms in biofilms have been shown to stimulate antibody production, but the humoral immune response is ineffective in killing biofilm-encased organisms.[12] The decreased susceptibility of sessile microorganisms to antimicrobial therapy is believed to be linked to multiple different pathways. Biofilms may act much like ion-exchange resins, and prevent the diffusion of certain antimicrobials to their target organisms.[12,13] Others have suggested that some subpopulations of sessile microorganisms enter a suppressed metabolic state, possibly from nutrient deprivation, and subsequently become non-susceptible to a variety of antimicrobials, especially those agents that are dependent on active microbial replication.[12]

Unfortunately from a clinical standpoint, traditional laboratory techniques have proved inadequate in biofilm-related infections.[15] Classic culture methods in microbiology are best suited for planktonic forms that grow well in conventional agar plates and broth. By contrast, as few as 1% of biofilm microorganisms grow via traditional laboratory culture methods; the application of molecular methods in aseptic loosening of prosthetic devices has found a large portion of these devices contaminated with bacteria. Also, standard laboratory methods may perform poorly in predicting antimicrobial susceptibilities for sessile forms of microorganisms, as their pattern of gene and protein expression differs from their planktonic forms. Consequently, treatment of biofilm-related infections may be directed against planktonic microorganisms that are easily identified while neglecting sessile organisms that are adherent to the device.[2] These sessile forms within biofilms often constitute a reservoir of microorganisms that persist even after antimicrobial therapy has eradicated the planktonic forms. These persistent forms are partly responsible for the high rate of treatment failure and relapse typically seen with implant infections.

RISK FACTORS AND MICROBIOLOGY

Potential routes for VGI include direct contamination at the time of initial surgery or during postoperative manipulation, retrograde infection resulting from superficial wound infection, or via hematogenous seeding. Infrainguinal revascularization proce-dures are much more likely than aortic grafts to become infected.[4] The presence of a groin incision is an especially important risk factor for infection.[4] Other commonly cited risk factors for VGI include diabetes mellitus, obesity, renal failure, revision surgery (particularly revision within 30 days), and use of prosthetic rather than native graft material (**Box 1**).[3,16–18] Prolonged operative time is also associated with infection.[3] Other investigators have reported a link between VGI and perioperative infection at another site, postoperative hyperglycemia, immunosuppression, and infected central lines.[4,19–22]

The lowest rates of infection following revascularization have been seen with anatomic, autologous reverse vein reconstructions.[4] For abdominal aortic grafts, endovascular repair does not appear to have a lower risk of infection than open repair; however, the risk of abdominal aortic graft infection is quite low with either approach.[22]

The most commonly isolated organisms in VGI are aerobic gram-positive cocci. In two series of more than 100 graft infections from 1972 to 1994, 22% of isolates were *S aureus*, 15% to 16% coagulase-negative staphylococci, and 18% were strepto-cocci.[7,23] Gram-negatives comprised 38% to 39% of all isolates, with *Pseudomonas* being the most common (18%).[4,7,23] Approximately one-third of VGI cases in these series were attributable to mixed gram-positive and gram-negative pathogens.[7,23] However, VGI microbiology has evolved, and other studies highlight a growing predominance of methicillin-resistant *S aureus* (MRSA).[24] Fungi and mycobacteria are rare but described causes of VGI.[25–28]

CLINICAL MANIFESTATIONS

VGI can present in myriad of ways, including inflammation or abscess surrounding the graft; exposure, erosion or fistulization of the graft; anastomotic disruption; and/or bacteremia, although clinically there is significant overlap among these syndromes. Infection of vascular grafts are often classified using the paradigm proposed by Samson: Grade 1, superficial, involving the skin and/or subcutaneous tissue; Grade 2, deep incisional, involving deep soft tissues, such as fascia and muscle including abscess cavities; Grade 3, infection without anastomosis site involvement; Grade 4, infection with anastomosis site involvement, but without anastomotic disruption; and Grade 5, infection with anastomotic disruption.[29]

Box 1
Risk factors for vascular graft infection
Presence of groin incision
Infrainguinal procedure
Wound-related complications (ie, hematoma, poor wound healing)
Comorbid conditions (diabetes mellitus, obesity, chronic renal insufficiency)
Revision surgery, especially within 30 days
Emergent surgery
Use of prosthetic graft
Prolonged operative time
Postoperative hyperglycemia
Perioperative infection at another site

Local signs of infection, such as cellulitis and wound drainage, are common and are often indistinguishable from superficial soft-tissue or surgical-incision infections. Occasionally bacteremia itself may be the only sign of VGI. Graft pseudoaneurysms can be seen in VGI but may also result from noninfectious mechanical failure. Specific signs and symptoms of VGI include abscess formation around the graft, sinus tract formation, septic emboli, frank graft exposure, and failure of the graft to incorporate into the surrounding soft tissue. A finding specific to aortic graft infection is aortoenteric fistula, which can be the presenting sign in about 30% of such infections.[30]

Systemic symptoms, such as fevers, leukocytosis, and sepsis, are much more variable. In one series, 35% of patients had only vague symptoms.[20] As a general rule, VGI with virulent organisms, such as S aureus, can be expected to present more rapidly with significant local and systemic findings, whereas VGI with less virulent organisms such as coagulase-negative staphylococci is more indolent and often lacks pronounced inflammatory changes.[31] Pounds and colleagues[4] reported that two-thirds of VGIs following revascularization procedures involved the graft body and/or anastomosis. The rate of anastomotic rupture can be greater than 20%,[4] and infection with highly virulent organisms (Pseudomonas and S aureus) predispose to anastomotic disruption.[1,4]

AVHG infections can present as isolated bacteremia, with typical findings expected of a surgical-site infection (SSI), or with draining sinus tracts or frank graft exposure without florid inflammatory findings.[5] AVHG infections can also present as silent infection, especially in abandoned, thrombosed grafts. This condition is well illustrated in the review by Nassar and Ayus[32] of hemodialysis patients with abandoned, nonfunctional AVHGs who developed fever or sepsis without overt localizing signs. Bacteremia was present in 15 of 20 patients with fever; indium scanning and surgical explantation confirmed frank infection in all 20 grafts. Among 21 asymptomatic controls, 15 were also indium scan positive; 13 of these subsequently were found to have frank purulence surrounding their old grafts. These results highlight the need for a high index of suspicion with AVHG infections.

DIAGNOSIS

Although VGI may be evident when frankly exposed graft or a sinus fistula is present, typically the diagnosis can often be more subtle because the clinical manifestations tend to be nonspecific. Laboratory findings may be helpful (leukocytosis, elevated inflammatory markers, or positive blood cultures), but are neither sensitive nor specific.[31] Overall, computed tomography (CT) is considered the best imaging modality. Specific CT findings that suggest infection include fluid surrounding the graft, especially with associated fat stranding and gas, lack of fat between graft and bowel (for aortic grafts), and anastomotic aneurysms.[33] Perigraft fluid is not an entirely specific finding, as sterile fluid can be found up to 3 months following graft placement, but an increase in the size of these fluid collections or persistence of such fluid beyond 3 months suggests infection.[34] The presence of gas around the graft is very common within the first week after surgery; however, persistence beyond 4 weeks postoperatively suggests infection.[34] The sensitivity of CT for advanced graft infections approaches 100%, but when low-grade infections are included the overall sensitivity is 55% and specificity is 100%.

Magnetic resonance imaging (MRI) likely has similar sensitivity and specificity to CT, but suffers from motion artifact and also cannot reliably distinguish between infected and noninfected fluid. Uninfected periprosthetic fluid collections may be seen on MRI for up to 6 months postoperatively. Finally, unlike CT, MRI does not allow for interventions, such as fluid aspiration. Despite these limitations, MRI can often be useful especially among patients with inconclusive CT results. By offering a noninvasive means to characterize vascular anatomy, magnetic resonance angiography is another way to evaluate the integrity of vascular grafts.

Indium-labeled white blood cell scintigraphy (WBC scans) may be an alternative diagnostic tool, but the sensitivity of such testing may be inferior (60%–100%) and studies are likely to be false-positive for several weeks postoperatively.[33,34] One potential advantage of WBC scanning is that contrast is not required, so the risk of nephrotoxicity is eliminated. Fluoroscopy has little role in the diagnosis of VGI, but sinography and angiography may help guide subsequent surgical therapy.[34] Many patients ultimately require a combination of imaging modalities, especially those with clinically challenging presentations.

Aspiration of perigraft fluid collections can be valuable,[35] though negative cultures or Gram stains do not rule out infection. As already noted, the sensitivity of conventional microbiology techniques may be poor for biofilm-related infections.[15] Molecular diagnostics techniques, while much more sensitive, have yet to achieve commercial viability or widespread use.

CLINICAL MANAGEMENT
General Principles

The treatment of VGI is challenging, due to both the inherently poor baseline health of these patient populations and the persistent nature of foreign-body infections. Management involves a combined approach, including extended courses of antimicrobial therapy along with surgical intervention that may involve of debridement of infected periprosthetic tissues, secondary revascularization, and possible excision of the infected device. The aggressiveness of surgical management will be dependent on multiple factors, including comorbid medical conditions, graft integrity, vascular anatomy, and the pathogen(s) involved.

Purely from an infectious disease standpoint, it would be ideal if the infected prosthetic graft could be removed, as such infections are rarely successfully sterilized with antimicrobial therapy alone and can serve as a reservoir for infection relapse.[10] However, from a surgical perspective this approach is often suboptimal or infeasible. In select cases, subtotal graft excision or even complete graft preservation may be possible. As a rule, graft infections associated with systemic sepsis or involvement of anastomoses, especially proximal anastomotic sites, mandate complete graft removal.[7,36] In situations with intact anastomoses but occluded grafts, subtotal excision of the occluded portion with oversewing of graft patch remnants to maintain patency of the artery can be attempted. Complete graft preservation is appropriate when the patient is not septic, the graft is patent, and the anastomoses are intact.[7]

In a 20-year series of VGI among 120 patients, Calligaro and colleagues[7] reported 12% mortality, 13% amputation, and successful complete or partial graft preservation in 71% and 85%, respectively.[7] These results compared favorably with other series having reported mortality rates of 9% to 36% and amputation rates of 27% to 79%. A potential disadvantage of graft-preserving approaches is the higher risk of relapse of infection, which may be as high as 82% as opposed to a 13% rate for complete graft excision.[10] Complete graft preservation is most likely to be successful with early-onset VGIs (<2 months after implantation).[36,37] Infection with *Pseudomonas* or MRSA are associated with higher rates of treatment failure and amputation.[11,36,37]

Options for revascularization include extra-anatomic and in situ approaches. For extra-anatomic bypass, the revascularization procedure is typically performed first and is then followed later by graft excision and debridement. In situ bypass is performed as a single procedure, and can involve the use of autogenous or allograft tissue or prosthetic grafts.[38] In situ approaches are typically associated with lower risk of amputation but higher rate of reinfection.[38,39] Lower rates of reinfection can be expected with the use of natural tissue as opposed to prosthetic material; patency rates are also improved.[16,38] It has been suggested that rifampin-impregnated prosthetic grafts may be equivalent in terms of reinfection rates in comparison with other modalities,[39] but a recent meta-analysis suggests that these rates are in fact higher than those for extra-anatomic bypass, cryopreserved allografts, and autogenous vein grafts.[38] Extra-anatomic bypass and complete graft excision classically has been considered the gold standard in the treatment of VGI, but a recent review suggests that for selected patients, in situ bypass can achieve equivalent or superior results to extra-anatomic bypass.[38]

An important adjunct to surgical therapy is aggressive management of wound care and potential dead space, which has traditionally involved vascularized tissue flaps to provide coverage of infected grafts. Such flaps can decrease mortality and amputation rates and increase the likelihood of graft salvage. The sartorius muscle tends to be the preferred choice for muscle flap given its proximity to the groin and ease of harvest, though it is susceptible to flap failure given its relatively tenuous blood supply and possible proximity to active groin infection.[36,40] Other muscle options for coverage include the gracilis, rectus femoral, rectus abdominis, gastrocnemius, soleus, tensor fascia lata, and omentum. The benefits of such flaps include superior management of potential wound dead space; improved healing time; and enhanced delivery of oxygen, antimicrobials, and phagocytes.[36] Nonrandomized studies suggest a reduction in amputation rates to below 30% and mortality rates to 0% to 14% compared with respective rates of 8% to 52% and 4% to 36% in the preflap era.[36] Vacuum-assisted closure (VAC) or negative pressure therapy (NPT) has emerged as an important modality for wound management. Dosluoglu and colleagues[41] reported graft salvage rates of 90% using VAC therapy for early-onset (>30 days) groin infections of Samson Grade 2 to 5.

Aortic Grafts

Although rare, infections of aortic grafts are potentially disastrous. The rate of VGI following aortic grafts has generally been reported as between 1% and 3%,[2] though one recent series reports a 7% rate following aortofemoral revascularization.[4] Groin incisions remain a major risk factor, and the rate of postoperative infection is higher for aortofemoral grafts than for aortoiliac grafts.[30] The rate of graft infection for completely intracavitary abdominal grafts is 0.44%.[22] The time of onset of aortic graft infection can be variable. One series reported the time of presentation from 1 to 84 months postsurgery (median 16 months).[42] Another series had a median time of onset of 67 months, with the longest interval being 20 years.[43]

The mortality rate is very high for early-onset (<30 days) aortic graft infection (>80%), whereas the survival rate for late-onset infections is much better (>70%).[30] The presence of enteral bleeding also predicts a high mortality rate.[30] The amputation rate following aortic graft infection has been reported at 10% to 25%.[44]

Manifestations of aortic graft infection include the typical signs and symptoms expected with SSIs, though malaise, fevers, and sepsis surprisingly are uncommon (6.3%–37%).[30,43,45] A palpable abdominal or groin mass is found in 23% to 44% of patients while inguinal swelling, wound infection, or fistulization can be seen in 40% to 59% of cases.[30,43] Enteral bleeding can be found in up to 31% of aortic graft infection, primarily with late-onset infection.[30]

The diagnosis of aortic graft infection can sometimes be made on clinical grounds when specific physical examination findings (eg, fistulization) are present, but often it is difficult to distinguish a simple SSI from a more insidious process. Routine blood work is of limited value, with the exception of blood cultures. The best diagnostic modality is CT, which has a sensitivity of 94% and a specificity of 85% for high-grade infections (using findings of perigraft fluid, perigraft soft-tissue attenuation, ectopic gas, pseudoaneurysm, or focal bowel wall thickening).[34] However, CT is less useful for low-grade infections. The overall sensitivity is 55% and specificity 100% for all cases of aortic graft infections.[34] Endoscopy is an insensitive modality for diagnosing aortoenteric fistula, providing the diagnosis in only 55% of cases.[30]

Management options for aortic graft infections vary from complete excision of the graft to more conservative approaches (**Fig. 1**). The optimal approach has not been

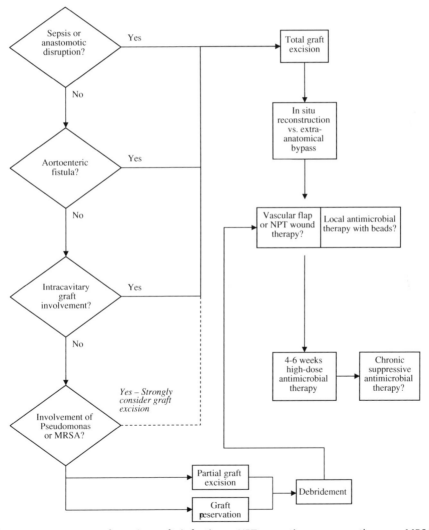

Fig. 1. Management of aortic graft infections. NPT, negative pressure therapy; MRSA, methicillin-resistant *Staphylococcus aureus*.

determined, and treatment of these serious infections is limited by the lack of large controlled trials. The classic approach to aortic graft infection has been complete graft removal with extra-anatomic bypass through an uninfected site via simultaneous or staged procedures.[42] Although this is still considered the gold standard in management, the drawbacks of this approach are significant and include increased surgical burden, high rates of mortality and amputation, and risk of aortic stump rupture.[38] Total or subtotal graft preservation can be attempted in selected patients provided there is not systemic sepsis, intracavitary involvement, anastomotic involvement, or infection with *Pseudomonas*.[44]

Other surgical options include debridement of infected tissue with in situ reconstruction using autogenous veins, cryopreserved allograft, or antimicrobial-coated synthetic grafts (primarily rifampin or silver).[38] A recent meta-analysis by O'Connor and colleagues[38] found that in situ reconstruction was superior to extra-anatomic bypass when considering early and late mortality, amputation, reinfection, and conduit failure. Rifampin-bonded prostheses had fewer amputations and conduit failures, and less early mortality but higher reinfection rate than any other modality. Autogenous vein reconstruction had the lowest rate of reinfection, and the lowest rate of late mortality was seen with autogenous and cryopreserved allografts. Because of these and other benefits, the femoral vein is being used more frequently for autogenous reconstruction and is emerging as the preferred approach at many institutions. Even so, there are also disadvantages for autogenous veins, including prolonged operative time and potential complications of vein harvesting. Cryopreserved grafts have unique limitations as well, including decreased durability as compared with prosthetic grafts and limited range of size, shape, and diameter. This meta-analysis did not include studies of silver-coated prosthetic grafts, as clinical experience with these devices remains limited. Overall, the rate of recurrent infection can be expected to be between 10% and 20%.[43]

For those patients who are extremely ill, percutaneous drainage of perigraft fluid can be attempted as a temporizing measure. One small series showed improved outcomes for patients managed with percutaneous drainage followed by definitive surgical intervention versus surgery alone.[46] However, it should be cautioned that the number of patients in this study was very small and there is an inherent selection bias in terms of which patients are deemed surgical candidates.

Local delivery of antimicrobials has been shown in vivo to reduce the numbers of bacteria in biofilms.[47] However, while some report good results using antibiotic-impregnated beads as adjunctive therapy for the treatment of VGI,[48] controlled trials demonstrating a definitive benefit are lacking. For selected patients who are not good surgical candidates, conservative therapy with antimicrobials alone may be an appropriate option. However, this approach is associated with an increased risk of mortality.[49]

Endovascular aneurysm repair (EVAR) is a relatively new approach to managing aortic aneurysms, with a primary advantage of decreased short-term surgical morbidity and mortality but at the cost of decreased durability.[50] The risk of endograft infection is rare (0.2%–0.7%), as such clinical experience with infection is limited.[51] Roughly one-third each of endograft infection cases presents as aortoenteric fistula, low-grade sepsis (eg, malaise, minimal symptoms), or severe sepsis.[51] In a recent series of 9 patients with endograft infection, the median time of presentation following EVAR was 33 months (range 6–80 months).[52]

The optimal management of endograft infection is unclear. One retrospective study suggested no significant difference in mortality for conservative therapy versus surgical therapy,[53] but this study was limited by small numbers. Ducasse and colleagues[54] reported a larger series with a mortality rate of 36.4% for aortic stent graft infections managed conservatively versus 14% for those managed surgically; the overall mortality was 18%. Laser and colleagues[52] recently reported their experience with 9 endograft infections. Eight of these patients were treated with endograft removal; 1 patient died of sepsis. Roughly equal numbers were treated with extra-anatomic bypass and in situ bypass; 7 of 9 patients (78%) were alive at 11 months.[52] All survivors received 4 to 6 weeks of postreconstruction antimicrobial therapy, and 5 of 7 survivors were placed on lifelong suppressive antimicrobial therapy.

Peripheral Grafts

The rate of infection following infrainguinal vascular grafts ranges from 1% to 6%.[55] While the incidence of infection remains low the potential morbidity and mortality is significant, with reported amputations rates of 8% to 52% and death rates of 14% to 58%.[3] As with aortic graft infections, the time to onset of infection following revascularization varies wildly. One series reported a median interval of 3 months postsurgery (range 0–187 months) before onset of infection.[10] The most common finding of infrainguinal VGI is wound drainage or the presence of a sinus tract (74%) followed by bleeding or pseudoaneurysm (40%), induration or tenderness (34%), systemic symptoms (eg, fevers, chills; 29%), and graft exposure (18%). Diagnostic modalities for peripheral VGI are similar to those for aortic graft infections.

Surgical management of peripheral graft infections can be divided into total excision of the implant with either extra-anatomic or in situ bypass, partial excision, or complete retention of the prosthesis (**Fig. 2**).[55] The choice of surgical modality largely depends on the extent of graft involvement. As a general rule, Samson Grade 1 wound infection can be managed with short courses of intravenous antimicrobial therapy while Grade 2 infections can be managed with local debridement and antimicrobials. Grade 3 or greater infections, that is, those involving the graft, typically will require either partial or total graft excision. The decision to retain any portion of the infected graft should be made with caution.

Mertens and colleagues[10] reported in a series of 68 patients a reoperation rate of 82% for continued sepsis for partial excision or complete retention of graft with in situ reconstruction, compared with 13% for complete graft excision with ex situ reconstruction. A caveat to this series is that only either Dacron or homograft was used for in situ reconstruction and not autogenous or antimicrobial-coated prostheses. These investigators also reported a postoperative mortality rate of 18%, more than half related to uncontrolled sepsis, in patients for whom limb salvage was attempted.

Others have reported better results with graft-preserving approaches provided the patients are carefully selected.[7] Long-term graft preservation was achieved in 71% of cases of complete graft preservation and in 85% of cases treated with partial graft preservation, provided patients did not have anastomotic disruption, graft occlusion, or systemic sepsis. Important adjunctive therapy in this series included repeated and aggressive debridement of the wound and graft as needed, and antiseptic wound dressing soaked with povidone-iodine or antimicrobials 3 times a day until healthy granulation tissue covered the anastomosis. Soft-tissue flaps were also aggressively used, and parenteral antimicrobials were given for at least 6 weeks. The mortality and amputation rates in this series were an impressive 12% and 4%, respectively. These same investigators also reported that involvement of *Pseudomonas* independently predicted salvage failure. Other investigators have found that involvement of MRSA has a higher rate of amputation and graft failure.[11] Of interest, using a similar protocol for successful graft preservation appears as likely with prosthetic or vein graft.[40] For those who fail graft preservation or have one of the contraindications noted

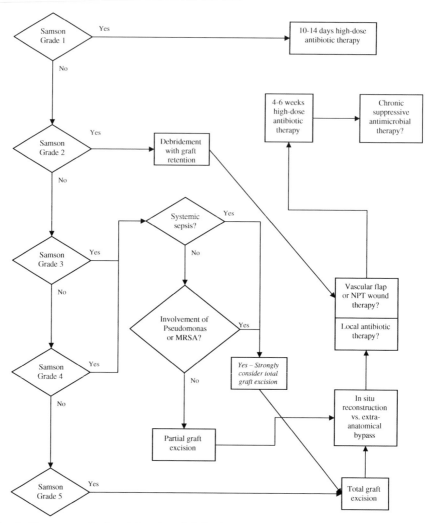

Fig. 2. Management of peripheral graft infections. NPT, negative pressure therapy; MRSA, methicillin-resistant *Staphylococcus aureus*.

(anastomotic disruption, sepsis, involvement of *Pseudomonas*, and possibly MRSA), complete graft excision with revascularization through an uninfected site is recommended.[7,55]

Hemodialysis Grafts

AVHGs are among the most commonly performed vascular procedures, with an estimated 250,000 individuals in the United States who require hemodialysis.[5] The rate of prosthetic AVHG infection is approximately 3% to 6%.[5,56] After thrombosis, infection is the most common complication of AVHG. Infectious complications, including AVHG infection, are associated with significant morbidity and play a role in at least one-quarter of all deaths of dialysis patients. AVHG infections can present at the site of prior surgical incision or at the site of cannulation for hemodialysis. Another common presentation is exposed graft or sinus tract, which was present in nearly half of the cases in one large series.[5] Other presenting signs included purulent drainage, sepsis, erythema, hemorrhage/hematoma, and pain.

The approach to surgical management of AVHG depends on the extent of graft involvement and severity of sepsis (**Fig. 3**).[5] Purulent involvement of the entire graft with anastomotic disruption or systemic sepsis generally warrants total graft removal. For stable individuals with total graft involvement but an intact, uninfected, well-incorporated anastomosis, subtotal graft excision (SGE), which retains an oversewn stump of the prosthesis on the originating artery, is typically appropriate. For cases in which only a segment of the graft is infected, partial graft excision (PGE), which involves limited removal of only the infected portion of the graft with segmental reconstruction through uninfected tissue, can be performed. The major advantage of SGE and PGE is maintenance of the patency of the originating artery and avoidance of a potentially morbid dissection. A major drawback of graft-sparing techniques is the potential for persistence of infection in the retained portion of graft. Schild and colleagues[57] reported in their large series that 17% of operative cases for infection in AVHG had previously infected AVHGs that were not completely removed. However, with careful selection of cases with well-incorporated graft remnants and aggressive

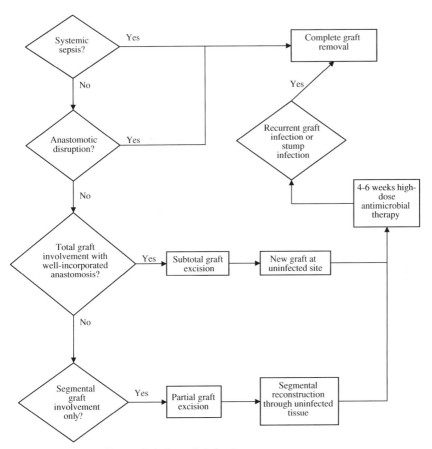

Fig. 3. Management of hemodialysis graft infections.

resection of obviously infected portions of the AVHG, recurrence of infection can be minimized.[5]

Antimicrobial Therapy

Antimicrobial therapy for VGI is best guided by intraoperative cultures. The accuracy of Gram stain alone is only 25%, therefore initial empiric therapy should include coverage for MRSA and *Pseudomonas*.[23] Vancomycin, linezolid, or daptomycin provide appropriate gram-positive coverage (MRSA, coagulase-negative staphlylococci, enterococci), and anti-Pseudomonal β-lactams, such as ceftazidime, cefepime, piperacillin-tazobactam, and ticarcillin-clavulanate, offer broad gram-negative coverage. Once cultures results are available, the regimen should be narrowed. For VGI involving staphylococci whereby the implant cannot be completely removed, the addition of rifampin as adjunctive therapy may improve outcomes, as has been demonstrated with staphylococcal orthopedic implant infections.[58] Similarly, for VGI with retained implant involving gram-negative organisms, the addition of a fluoroquinolone may be beneficial.[59]

There are no randomized controlled trials to define the optimal length of antimicrobial therapy, but most experts recommend extended courses of parenteral agents, for example, 4 to 6 weeks.[7,55] Certain patients may be candidates for chronic, possibly lifelong, suppressive therapy, especially if the infected graft cannot be completely excised.[52,60,61]

Antimicrobials are not therapeutically neutral, and the decision to initiate therapy should not be made lightly. The incidence of adverse drug reactions is increased with prolonged use. These side effects may be simple, such as diarrhea or rash, but one series reported rates of myelosuppression of 16% and nephrotoxicity of 8%.[62] Access-related problems occurred in 9% to 11% of patients, including an infection and line-related thrombosis rate of 2% each for patients with peripherally inserted central catheters.[62]

PREVENTION

The principles of prevention of VGI are no different to those for the prevention of SSI in general: proper preoperative patient preparation, careful surgical technique and antisepsis, hand washing, timely administration of preoperative antibiotic prophylaxis, and meticulous wound care.[63,64] In addition, careful control of blood sugars, oxygenation, and body temperature during the perioperative period also appear to decrease the risk of SSI.

Preoperative antimicrobial prophylaxis should be administered 30 to 60 minutes before the procedure if a first-generation or second-generation cephalosporin is used. For institutions with high rates of MRSA or for a patient known to be a carrier of MRSA, daptomycin or vancomycin can be administered adjunctively. If vancomycin is used, it should be given 60 to 120 minutes before surgery. For procedures longer than 3 hours, additional doses of cephalosporins should be administered if these are the prophylaxis agents being used. Antimicrobial prophylaxis longer than 24 hours does not have any additional benefit.[65] A recent meta-analysis of SSI prevention trials in vascular surgery found that prophylactic antimicrobial therapy reduced the risk of wound and graft infection.[65] Rifampin-bonded Dacron grafts did not reduce the short-term or long-term risk of graft infection. There was also no benefit to suction wound drainage, preoperative washes with chlorhexidine or povidone-iodine, minimally invasive techniques, intraoperative glove changes, or varying methods of wound closure.

Nasal carriage of *S aureus*, in particular MRSA, has been shown to increase the risk of early SSI greater than eightfold.[63] Unfortunately, the data for *S aureus* decolonization for prevention of SSI is mixed. Intranasal mupirocin alone does not appear to reduce the risk of SSI,[66,67] which may be in large part due to the carriage of *S aureus* at extranasal sites. Recently, a randomized control trial using intranasal mupirocin plus chlorhexidine washes demonstrated a reduced risk (RR = 0.21) of SSI with *S aureus*.[68]

SUMMARY

VGIs remain a devastating health problem that imposes a high risk of amputation and mortality for the individual patient plus high costs on the health care system in general. The best treatment modalities for such infections have yet to be determined. Surgical interventions continue to play a key role in terms of definitive source control and limb preservation, and recent years have seen a movement toward graft-conserving techniques that show great promise in reduction of mortality and morbidity. Antimicrobial prophylaxis will continue to play an important part in preoperative prevention of and treatment of VGI. The optimal length of antimicrobial therapy and the value of prolonged suppressive treatment remain undefined. Understanding of the pathogenesis of biofilm-related infections and the development of rapid molecular diagnostic techniques may ultimately provide revolutionary insights into the prevention and treatment of these infections.

REFERENCES

1. Wilson SE. New alternatives in management of the infected vascular prosthesis. Surg Infect (Larchmt) 2001;2:171–5.
2. Herscu G, Wilson SE. Prosthetic infection: lessons from treatment of the infected vascular graft. Surg Clin North Am 2009;89:391–401.
3. Chang JK, Calligaro KD, Ryan S, et al. Risk factors associated with infection of lower extremity revascularization: analysis of 365 procedures performed at a teaching hospital. Ann Vasc Surg 2003;17:91–6.
4. Pounds LL, Montes-Walters M, Mayhall CG, et al. A changing pattern of infection after major vascular reconstructions. Vasc Endovascular Surg 2005;39:511–7.
5. Ryan SV, Calligaro KD, Scharff J, et al. Management of infected prosthetic dialysis arteriovenous grafts. J Vasc Surg 2004;39:73–8.
6. Darouiche RO. Treatment of infections associated with surgical implants. N Engl J Med 2004;350:1422–9.
7. Calligaro KD, Veith FJ, Schwartz ML, et al. Selective preservation of infected prosthetic arterial grafts. Analysis of a 20-year experience with 120 extracavitary-infected grafts. Ann Surg 1994;220:461–9.
8. Edwards WH Jr, Martin RS 3rd, Jenkins JM, et al. Primary graft infections. J Vasc Surg 1987;6:235–9.
9. Jensen LJ, Kimose HH. Prosthetic graft infections: a review of 720 arterial prosthetic reconstructions. Thorac Cardiovasc Surg 1985;33:389–91.
10. Mertens RA, O'Hara PJ, Hertzer NR, et al. Surgical management of infrainguinal arterial prosthetic graft infections: review of a thirty-five-year experience. J Vasc Surg 1995;21:782–90.
11. Taylor MD, Napolitano LM. Methicillin-resistant *Staphylococcus aureus* infections in vascular surgery: increasing prevalence. Surg Infect (Larchmt) 2004;5:180–7.
12. Costerton JW, Stewart PS, Greenberg EP. Bacterial biofilms: a common cause of persistent infections. Science 1999;284:1318–22.

13. Schierholz JM, Beuth J. Implant infections: a haven for opportunistic bacteria. J Hosp Infect 2001;49:87–93.
14. Zimmerli W, Waldvogel FA, Vaudaux P, et al. Pathogenesis of foreign body infection: description and characteristics of an animal model. J Infect Dis 1982;146: 487–97.
15. Costerton JW, Post JC, Ehrlich GD, et al. New methods for the detection of orthopedic and other biofilm infections. FEMS Immunol Med Microbiol 2011;61: 133–40.
16. Calligaro KD, Syrek JR, Dougherty MJ, et al. Use of arm and lesser saphenous vein compared with prosthetic grafts for infrapopliteal arterial bypass: are they worth the effort? J Vasc Surg 1997;26:919–24.
17. Lee ES, Santilli SM, Olson MM, et al. Wound infection after infrainguinal bypass operations: multivariate analysis of putative risk factors. Surg Infect (Larchmt) 2000;1:257–63.
18. Pedersen G, Laxdal E, Hagala M, et al. Local infections after above-knee prosthetic femoropopliteal bypass for intermittent claudication. Surg Infect (Larchmt) 2004;5:174–9.
19. Antonios VS, Noel AA, Steckelberg JM, et al. Prosthetic vascular graft infection: a risk factor analysis using a case-control study. J Infect 2006;53:49–55.
20. Fiorani P, Speziale F, Calisti A, et al. Endovascular graft infection: preliminary results of an international enquiry. J Endovasc Ther 2003;10:919–27.
21. Vriesendorp TM, Morelis QJ, Devries JH, et al. Early post-operative glucose levels are an independent risk factor for infection after peripheral vascular surgery. A retrospective study. Eur J Vasc Endovasc Surg 2004;28:520–5.
22. Vogel TR, Symons R, Flum DR. The incidence and factors associated with graft infection after aortic aneurysm repair. J Vasc Surg 2008;47:264–9.
23. Calligaro KD, Veith FJ, Schwartz ML, et al. Recommendations for initial antibiotic treatment of extracavitary arterial graft infections. Am J Surg 1995;170:123–5.
24. Nasim A, Thompson MM, Naylor AR, et al. The impact of MRSA on vascular surgery. Eur J Vasc Endovasc Surg 2001;22:211–4.
25. Collazos J, Mayo J, Martinez E, et al. Prosthetic vascular graft infection due to Aspergillus species: case report and literature review. Eur J Clin Microbiol Infect Dis 2001;20:414–7.
26. Lephart P, Ferrieri P, van Burik JA. Reservoir of Candida albicans infection in a vascular bypass graft demonstrates a stable karyotype over six months. Med Mycol 2004;42:255–60.
27. Matthay RA, Levin DC, Wicks AB, et al. Disseminated histoplasmosis involving an aortofemoral prosthetic graft. JAMA 1976;235:1478–9.
28. Raffetto JD, Bernardo J, Menzoian JO. Aortobifemoral graft infection with Mycobacterium tuberculosis: treatment with abscess drainage, debridement, and long-term administration of antibiotic agents. J Vasc Surg 2004;40:826–9.
29. Zetrenne E, McIntosh BC, McRae MH, et al. Prosthetic vascular graft infection: a multi-center review of surgical management. Yale J Biol Med 2007;80:113–21.
30. Soetevent C, Klemm PL, Stalenhoef AF, et al. Vascular graft infection in aortoiliac and aortofemoral bypass surgery: clinical presentation, diagnostic strategies and results of surgical treatment. Neth J Med 2004;62:446–52.
31. FitzGerald SF, Kelly C, Humphreys H. Diagnosis and treatment of prosthetic aortic graft infections: confusion and inconsistency in the absence of evidence or consensus. J Antimicrob Chemother 2005;56:996–9.
32. Nassar GM, Ayus JC. Clotted arteriovenous grafts: a silent source of infection. Semin Dial 2000;13:1–3.

33. Orton DF, LeVeen RF, Saigh JA, et al. Aortic prosthetic graft infections: radiologic manifestations and implications for management. Radiographics 2000;20: 977–93.

34. Thomas P, Forstrom L. In-111 labeled purified granulocytes in the diagnosis of synthetic vascular graft infections. Clin Nucl Med 1994;19:1075–8.

35. Rossi P, Arata FM, Salvatori FM, et al. Prosthetic graft infection: diagnostic and therapeutic role of interventional radiology. J Vasc Interv Radiol 1997;8:271–7.

36. Seify H, Moyer HR, Jones GE, et al. The role of muscle flaps in wound salvage after vascular graft infections: the Emory experience. Plast Reconstr Surg 2006;117:1325–33.

37. Calligaro KD, Veith FJ, Schwartz ML, et al. Differences in early versus late extracavitary arterial graft infections. J Vasc Surg 1995;22:680–5.

38. O'Connor S, Andrew P, Batt M, et al. A systematic review and meta-analysis of treatments for aortic graft infection. J Vasc Surg 2006;44:38–45.

39. Young RM, Cherry KJ Jr, Davis PM, et al. The results of in situ prosthetic replacement for infected aortic grafts. Am J Surg 1999;178:136–40.

40. Calligaro KD, Veith FJ, Sales CM, et al. Comparison of muscle flaps and delayed secondary intention wound healing for infected lower extremity arterial grafts. Ann Vasc Surg 1994;8:31–7.

41. Dosluoglu HH, Schimpf DK, Schultz R, et al. Preservation of infected and exposed vascular grafts using vacuum assisted closure without muscle flap coverage. J Vasc Surg 2005;42:989–92.

42. Lehnert T, Gruber HP, Maeder N, et al. Management of primary aortic graft infection by extra-anatomic bypass reconstruction. Eur J Vasc Surg 1993;7:301–7.

43. Hart JP, Eginton MT, Brown KR, et al. Operative strategies in aortic graft infections: is complete graft excision always necessary? Ann Vasc Surg 2005;19:154–60.

44. Calligaro KD, Veith FJ. Graft preserving methods for managing aortofemoral prosthetic graft infection. Eur J Vasc Endovasc Surg 1997;14(Suppl A):38–42.

45. Menawat SS, Gloviczki P, Serry RD, et al. Management of aortic graft-enteric fistulae. Eur J Vasc Endovasc Surg 1997;14(Suppl A):74–81.

46. Belair M, Soulez G, Oliva VL, et al. Aortic graft infection: the value of percutaneous drainage. AJR Am J Roentgenol 1998;171:119–24.

47. Keeling WB, Myers AR, Stone PA, et al. Regional antibiotic delivery for the treatment of experimental prosthetic graft infections. J Surg Res 2009;157:223–6.

48. Stone PA, Armstrong PA, Bandyk DF, et al. Use of antibiotic-loaded polymethylmethacrylate beads for the treatment of extracavitary prosthetic vascular graft infections. J Vasc Surg 2006;44:757–61.

49. Saleem BR, Meerwaldt R, Tielliu IF, et al. Conservative treatment of vascular prosthetic graft infection is associated with high mortality. Am J Surg 2010;200:47–52.

50. Greenhalgh RM, Brown LC, Powell JT, et al. Endovascular versus open repair of abdominal aortic aneurysm. N Engl J Med 2010;362:1863–71.

51. Hobbs SD, Kumar S, Gilling-Smith GL. Epidemiology and diagnosis of endograft infection. J Cardiovasc Surg (Torino) 2010;51:5–14.

52. Laser A, Baker N, Rectenwald J, et al. Graft infection after endovascular abdominal aortic aneurysm repair. J Vasc Surg 2011;54(1):58–63.

53. Cernohorsky P, Reijnen MM, Tielliu IF, et al. The relevance of aortic endograft prosthetic infection. J Vasc Surg 2011;54(2):327–33.

54. Ducasse E, Calisti A, Speziale F, et al. Aortoiliac stent graft infection: current problems and management. Ann Vasc Surg 2004;18:521–6.

55. Zetrenne E, Wirth GA, McIntosh BC, et al. Managing extracavitary prosthetic vascular graft infections: a pathway to success. Ann Plast Surg 2006;57:677–82.

56. Nassar GM, Ayus JC. Infectious complications of the hemodialysis access. Kidney Int 2001;60:1–13.

57. Schild AF, Simon S, Prieto J, et al. Single-center review of infections associated with 1,574 consecutive vascular access procedures. Vasc Endovascular Surg 2003;37:27–31.

58. Zimmerli W, Widmer AF, Blatter M, et al. Role of rifampin for treatment of orthopedic implant-related staphylococcal infections: a randomized controlled trial. Foreign-Body Infection (FBI) Study Group. JAMA 1998;279:1537–41.

59. Martinez-Pastor JC, Munoz-Mahamud E, Vilchez F, et al. Outcome of acute prosthetic joint infections due to gram-negative bacilli treated with open debridement and retention of the prosthesis. Antimicrob Agents Chemother 2009;53:4772–7.

60. Terpling S, Schade Larsen C, Schonheyder HC. Long-term home-based parenteral antibiotic treatment of a prosthetic vascular graft infection caused by *Pseudomonas aeruginosa*. Scand J Infect Dis 2006;38:388–92.

61. Mussa FF, Hedayati N, Zhou W, et al. Prevention and treatment of aortic graft infection. Expert Rev Anti Infect Ther 2007;5:305–15.

62. Hoffman-Terry ML, Fraimow HS, Fox TR, et al. Adverse effects of outpatient parenteral antibiotic therapy. Am J Med 1999;106:44–9.

63. Bandyk DF. Vascular surgical site infection: risk factors and preventive measures. Semin Vasc Surg 2008;21:119–23.

64. Anderson DJ, Kaye KS, Classen D, et al. Strategies to prevent surgical site infections in acute care hospitals. Infect Control Hosp Epidemiol 2008;29(Suppl 1): S51–61.

65. Stewart A, Eyers PS, Earnshaw JJ. Prevention of infection in arterial reconstruction. Cochrane Database Syst Rev 2006;3:CD003073.

66. Coates T, Bax R, Coates A. Nasal decolonization of *Staphylococcus aureus* with mupirocin: strengths, weaknesses and future prospects. J Antimicrob Chemother 2009;64:9–15.

67. Robicsek A, Beaumont JL, Thomson RB Jr, et al. Topical therapy for methicillin-resistant *Staphylococcus aureus* colonization: impact on infection risk. Infect Control Hosp Epidemiol 2009;30:623–32.

68. Bode LG, Kluytmans JA, Wertheim HF, et al. Preventing surgical-site infections in nasal carriers of *Staphylococcus aureus*. N Engl J Med 2010;362:9–17.

Cardiovascular Implantable Electronic Device Associated Infections

Tejal Gandhi, MD[a],*, Thomas Crawford, MD[b],
James Riddell IV, MD[a]

KEYWORDS

- Cardiovascular implantable electronic devices • Infection
- Management

There is a high incidence of cardiovascular disease among the United States' population and, subsequently, an increasing number of patients undergoing placement of cardiovascular implantable electronic devices (CIEDs) to improve quality of life and survival. The incidence of cardiovascular disease is highest among older adults and, consequently, recent population-based studies suggest that the mean age at CIED placement exceeds 70 years.[1,2] Based on large clinical trials, the American College of Cardiology and the American Heart Association (AHA) have issued guidelines with expanded indications for use of implantable cardioverter-defibrillators (ICDs) for primary prevention of sudden cardiac death and biventricular pacemakers (PPMs) for symptomatic improvement in patients with heart failure.[3,4] As a result, use of CIED has increased in the United States and worldwide.[5–7]

The management of CIED infections is clinically challenging and it results in substantial morbidity and mortality for patients.[8] This article presents an overview of cardiac device infections, including current epidemiology and specific host and procedural risk factors for the development of CIED infections. The microbiology will also be reviewed with a focus on both common and unusual pathogens. Finally, recent advances in the diagnosis and the multifaceted approach essential to successful management of CIED infection are considered.

The authors have nothing to disclose.
[a] Division of Infectious Diseases, University of Michigan Medical School, 3119 Taubman Center, 1500 East Medical Center Drive, SPC 5378, Ann Arbor, MI 48109, USA
[b] Division of Cardiovascular Medicine, Cardiovascular Center, University of Michigan Medical School, 1500 East Medical Center Drive, SPC 5856, Ann Arbor, MI 48109, USA
* Corresponding author.
E-mail address: tgandhi@med.umich.edu

Infect Dis Clin N Am 26 (2012) 57–76
doi:10.1016/j.idc.2011.09.001
0891-5520/12/$ – see front matter © 2012 Elsevier Inc. All rights reserved.

id.theclinics.com

EPIDEMIOLOGY AND RISK FACTORS

When ICDs were first used in the 1980s, these devices were generally implanted by cardiac surgeons with the assistance of cardiologists.[9] At that time, procedures were quite complex because the large generators required implantation within the abdomen and tunneled leads were placed epicardially via thoracotomy. Infection rates using this approach were reported as high as 17%.[10] Over time, the generator size has decreased substantially, facilitating implantation in the pectoral region and insertion of transvenous leads through the subclavian vein in a single procedure. One study reported long-term infection rates associated with subcutaneous pectoral implantation at 0.5%, compared with an infection rate of 3.5% for abdominal implantations.[11] Another center reported a similarly low infection rate of 0.2% with pectoral implantation.[12] A more recent study, which used data from the National Hospital Discharge Survey (NHDS), estimated that 4.1% to 5.8% of CIED devices became infected between 2004 and 2006.[8]

Multiple studies confirm increasing implantation rates but, surprisingly, rates of CIED infection have increased disproportionately (**Fig. 1**).[8,13] To illustrate, a study of Medicare beneficiaries found a 42% increase in cardiac device implantation from 1990 to 1999, but the infection rate increased from 0.94 device infections per 1000 beneficiaries to 2.11 per 1000, reflecting a 124% increase during the same 10-year period.[13] Similarly, a study that reviewed NHDS data reported a 57% increase in infections but only a 12% increase in devices implanted between 2004 and 2006 (see **Fig. 1**).[8] Overall, CIED infections rates range between 0.2% and 5.8% with pectoral implantation, but these rates have exceeded predictions. Although the exact reasons for this increase remain unknown, more device use among older patients and others with comorbid conditions may provide a partial explanation.[6,14]

Multiple studies have evaluated potential host and procedural risk factors for CIED infection.[2,8,15–18] A study examining 4856 patients who had either a PPM or a ICD device implanted found comorbid conditions such as heart failure, diabetes, renal insufficiency, and anticoagulation to be significant risk factors for the development of CIED infection.[15] Renal insufficiency (creatinine clearance ≤60 mL per minute) was highlighted as a particularly strong risk factor with a prevalence of 42% in patients with CIED infection compared with 13% of control patients (odds ratio [OR] 4.8; CI 2.1–10.7). Others have associated chronic renal insufficiency with increased risk of CIED infection[8] and as a risk factor for increased mortality among patients with

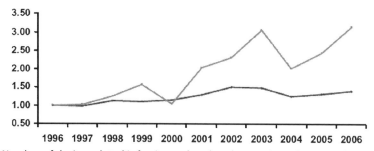

Fig. 1. Number of device-related infections related to the number of new implanted devices over time in the United States. (*purple line*) Number of infected implanted cardiac devices by year of hospitalization normalized to the year 1996. (*blue line*) Proportional increase in the number of devices implanted normalized to the year 1996. (*From* Voigt A, Shalaby A, Saba S. Rising rates of cardiac rhythm management device infections in the United States: 1996 through 2003. J Am Coll Cardiol 2006;48(3):590–1; with permission.)

a CIED.[19] Patients with end-stage renal disease who undergo hemodialysis are at risk for dialysis-access–associated bloodstream infection, which can result in secondary infection of intravascular components of the cardiac device. Additional host factors, such as chronic obstructive pulmonary disease,[17] corticosteroid use,[16] and advanced age (>60 years),[18] have also been identified as risk factors for CIED infection. The Prospective Evaluation of Pacemaker Lead Endocarditis (PEOPLE) study evaluated 6319 recipients of CIED from 44 medical centers.[2] Several risk factors previously identified in single-center studies, such as diabetes mellitus, advanced age, or receipt of oral anticoagulation, were not found to be associated with CIED infection in this large, prospective study.

In addition to host factors, CIED infection has been associated with several procedural and device-specific factors. Multiple studies have shown antimicrobial prophylaxis before PPM and ICD placement decreases the risk of CIED infection.[2,16–18,20] The presence of two pacing leads,[16] generator replacement,[18,21] temporary pacing before implantation,[2] fevers within 24 hours before implantation,[2] early reintervention for pocket hematoma or lead dislodgement,[2,21] development of postoperative complications at the generator pocket,[17,22] and presence of epicardial leads[17] have been identified as risk factors for CIED infection.

A recent study[17] showed an independent association between early infection and epicardial lead placement. The same study found that postoperative hematoma, wound dehiscence, delayed healing, and drainage from the pocket site were predictive of postoperative complications at the generator pocket. Prolonged hospitalization (≥2 days) after the procedure and chronic obstructive pulmonary disease were associated with late-onset infection. Another recent study sought to determine whether risk factors differed for a localized generator pocket infection compared with systemic infection.[18] The investigators found that more patients with localized pocket infection had undergone generator replacement (17%) versus those who developed systemic infection (10%). The presence of a central venous catheter was a strong risk factor for systemic infection (20%) compared with localized pocket infections (2%).

The type and complexity of the actual device CIED may also influence infection risk, but results are conflicting. For example, one group found a similar incidence of infection among patients with single chamber PPM system (0.82%) compared with dual chamber (1%),[23] but a similar study by a different group found that patients with dual chamber systems developed more infections.[24] Others have also reported that patients with more complex devices, such as dual-chamber or triple-chamber devices, were more likely to develop infection.[21] A recent, large, cohort study examining complication rates associated with PPM or ICD generator replacement and upgrade procedures found similar event rates for both major and minor infections among patients undergoing generator replacement and transvenous lead addition (1.1%) compared with patients who did not require lead addition (1.4%).[25] Other investigators have suggested that ICDs might carry an increased risk compared with PPM.[1,8]

In summary, the current literature on risk factors associated with CIED infection is mostly limited to single-center, retrospective studies with small numbers of patients. Larger, multicenter, prospective studies are essential to developing better risk-stratification paradigms. Such stratification would permit further study of targeted preventative interventions that, in turn, could reduce the risk of CIED infection.

MICROBIOLOGY

Gram-positive organisms remain the predominant pathogens associated with CIED infection—specifically coagulase-negative staphylococci (CNS) or *Staphylococcus aureus.*[17,18,26,27] A recent Mayo Clinic study examining CIED infections reported CNS in 41% of patients, *S aureus* in 41% of patients, and various gram-negative bacilli, fungi, and *Propionibacterium acnes* in the remainder.[26] A French study noted CNS in 36 out of 60 cases (60%), *S aureus* in 15%, and gram-negative bacteria or streptococcal species causing infection in the others.[27] In contrast, several studies have found *S aureus* more frequently than CNS in CIED infections.[21,28] Based on these reports, clinicians initiating empiric antimicrobial therapy for CIED infection should include coverage for methicillin resistant Staphylococcus spp while awaiting culture results.

Although CNS and *S aureus* are encountered most frequently, many case reports and case series describe unusual or atypical pathogens associated with CIED infection (**Table 1**). Gram-negative bacteria such as *Stenotrophomonas maltophilia,*[29] *Providencia rettgeri,*[30] *Achromobacter xylosoxidans,*[31] and *Burkholderia cepacia*[32] are reported to cause both pocket infections and CIED-associated endocarditis.

Although rare, a surprising number of case reports describe fungal infections of CIEDs, including Mucor spp,[33] Aspergillus,[26,34-37] Acremonium,[38,39] *Scedosporium prolificans,*[40] and *S apiospermum* (*Pseudallescheria boydii*).[41-43] Most patients with a fungal CIED infection were not immunocompromised; therefore, the most likely route of entry was during device placement. In addition, these patients seem to experience a high rate of systemic embolism and high mortality rates. Diagnosis is challenging because fungi (especially filamentous fungi) are rarely isolated from blood cultures. In most cases, a culture of the vegetation or purulent material within the pacer pocket or postmortem examination identified these pathogens.

Mycobacterium species are another uncommon but well-described pathogen in CIED infections. Pacemaker pocket-site infections with a newly recognized organism, *Mycobacterium goodii,* have been reported in the United States, France, and Japan.[44-46] Other rapidly growing atypical mycobacteria are also reported, such as *M fortuitum*[47-49] and *M abscessus.*[50,51] These organisms are commonly found in the environment and likely contaminate the device or pocket at the time of insertion or during surgical manipulation. Reactivation of *M tuberculosis* causing a CIED infection has also been identified in several case reports.[52-54]

The fact that such a wide range of organisms has been associated with cardiac device infections underscores the importance of accurately identifying the causative pathogens so that appropriate therapy can be administered. Cultures performed at the time of device removal should include mycobacterial and fungal culture in addition to routine bacterial cultures. When an atypical organism is suspected, tissue can also be submitted for polymerase chain reaction analysis.

DIAGNOSIS

Patients with cardiac device infections can be divided into two broad clinical categories. The first group has infection limited to the generator pocket site, with or without associated bacteremia. The second group has a primary endovascular infection with lead vegetations or an infection of intracardiac structures (endocarditis). Among patients who develop CIED infections, several studies have found that pocket infections occur more frequently than device-related endocarditis.[1,16-18,21,55] A single-center, retrospective review of 189 patients with CIED infections reported that 69% of patients had a generator pocket infection and 23% had a device-related endocarditis[16]; among patients with isolated generator pocket infection, 25% were found to have bacteremia.

Table 1
Organisms associated with infections of pacemakers or implantable cardioverter-defibrillator devices

Organism	Incidence	References
Gram-positive bacteria		
Coagulase-negative Staphylococcus	25%–72%	21,26–28,55
Staphylococcus aureus	15%–41%	21,26–28,55
Streptococcus sp	8%–20%	27,28
Enterococcus sp	—	26
Staphylococcus schleiferi	—	91
Propionibacterium acnes	—	26,95
Staphylococcus hominis	—	27
Bacillus cereus	—	96
Nocardia nova	—	97
Gram-negative bacteria		
Campylobacter fetus	—	98
Pseudomonas aeruginosa	—	26,99,100
Achromobacter xylosoxidans	—	26,31
Brucella melitensis	—	92–94
Klebsiella	—	27
Enterobacter	—	27
Stenotrophomonas	—	29
Providencia rettgeri	—	30
Burkholderia cepacia	—	32
Fungi		
Candida sp	—	26,101,102
Zygomycetes (*Mucor* spp)	—	33
Aspergillus fumigatus	—	26,34–37
Acremonium sp	—	38,39
Scedosporium apiospermum	—	42,43
Scedosporium prolificans	—	40,42
Mycobacteria		
M tuberculosis	—	52–54
M goodii	—	44–46
M fortuitum	—	47–49
M abscessus	—	50,51
M avium	—	103,104

The time to development of CIED infection varies among studies.[16,21,26,55,56] One retrospective study suggested that patients had a fairly even distribution with regard to the timing of infection, with 25% of patients developing infection within 0 to 28 days after device placement, 33% from 30 to 364 days after device placement, and 42% greater than 365 days after device placement.[55] In contrast, a Canadian study found that 60% of device infections developed within 3 months of the most recent intervention[21] and a large prospective study in France reported the median time to infection was 52 days (interquartile range 24–162 days).[2]

CIED infections can present with a wide variety of symptoms and can often pose a diagnostic challenge for clinicians. Typical signs or symptoms can include localized signs of inflammation at the generator pocket, such as erythema, warmth, fluctuance, wound dehiscence, tenderness, purulent drainage, or erosion of the generator or lead through the skin with or without associated localized inflammatory changes.[1,16,57,58] Studies have generally defined CIED-associated endocarditis by the presence of lead or valvular vegetations on echocardiography or by whether the modified Duke criteria for infective endocarditis are met.[1,18,26,58,59] In these studies, a vegetation has been defined as an oscillating intracardiac mass on the device leads, cardiac valve leaflets, or endocardial surface, confirmed by imaging in more than one echocardiographic plane and either a positive blood culture or lead tip culture.[18,26,58,60]

Several studies examining the clinical presentation of CIED infections have reported that localizing signs of inflammation occur more frequently than systemic symptoms.[16,18,55] For example, in a series of 123 patients with CIED infection, 69% of patients presented with only symptoms localized to the pulse generator pocket.[55] In another study of 189 patients, most had localizing inflammatory signs, but less than half presented with systemic symptoms.[16] Sohail and colleagues[16] also found 5% of patients had generator erosion without local inflammatory signs and that 11% of patients with purulence in their generator pocket during intraoperative exploration did not have inflammatory signs on physical examination. Several studies have also found that between 20% and 50% patients with bacteremia or CIED-associated endocarditis may not present with systemic signs of infection, such as fever, chills, malaise, or anorexia,[18,26,27,55] and between 27% to 65% will not have localized inflammatory signs at the generator pocket.[17,18,26,27,57] At times, persistent pain at the pocket site may be the only indication of a pocket infection.[61] The myriad of clinical presentations highlights the importance of clinicians maintaining a high index of suspicion for CIED infection even among patients without systemic symptoms or localizing inflammatory symptoms.

A recent scientific statement by the AHA on CIED infections and their management has provided formal guidance on the diagnosis of CIED infections.[62] For patients with suspected CIED infection, clinicians should perform two sets of blood cultures, tissue cultures from the generator pocket site, and cultures of the lead tips. A tissue culture from the generator pocket is more sensitive than a swab culture of the pocket and, thus, is the preferred culture method.[63] Most experts do not recommend percutaneous aspiration of the generator pocket because culture information can be obtained at the time of device extraction and aspiration places patients at risk for the introduction of skin flora into the pocket site if extraction is not performed.[62]

Blood cultures should be repeated after device explantation to confirm clearance of bacteremia and to assist in determining duration of antimicrobial therapy. In previous studies, blood cultures identified a causative pathogen in 33% to 40%[16,18,55] of all cases of CIED infection, and in 68.3% to 100% of cases with CIED-associated endocarditis.[16,18,26,27,56] Cultures of the generator pocket tissue and lead tip cultures have a higher likelihood of identifying the causative pathogen; generator pocket cultures identified a causative pathogen in 61% to 81%[16,26,55] and lead tip cultures were positive in 63.3% to 79%[26,27,55] of cases. Establishing the diagnosis of endocarditis by a positive lead culture without evidence of vegetation on transesophageal echocardiography or bacteremia can be misleading and inappropriately result in an extended duration of antimicrobial therapy.[26,62] In this clinical scenario, patients have successfully been treated for a pocket infection with a shorter duration of antimicrobial therapy.[26]

A transesophageal echocardiography (TEE) should be performed when patients are bacteremic, when endocarditis is suspected because of clinical findings, or when blood cultures are negative in the setting of recent antibiotic exposure. Caution should be exercised in cases of incidental masses associated with leads found in the absence of clinical suspicion for infection because many may be thrombotic in nature.[64] Clinicians should not rely on transthoracic echocardiography for ruling out endocarditis because of low sensitivity in comparison to TEE.[26,65]

MANAGEMENT OF CARDIAC DEVICE INFECTIONS

CIED infection is associated with substantial morbidity and mortality.[8,10,13,58] Among published studies, mortality ranges from 7.4% to 18%[55,66,67] with complete device extraction and from 8.4% to 41%[66,67] with partial device extraction or antimicrobial therapy alone. The approach to optimal management of CIED infections encompasses a combination of complete device extraction and appropriate antimicrobial therapy targeting the causative pathogens. Complete device extraction is recommended for generator or lead erosion (even without evidence of local inflammation), pocket infection, valve endocarditis, and lead endocarditis because antimicrobials alone or in combination with partial device removal is associated with unacceptably high relapse rates and significant mortality.[55,60,66,68] A superficial, localized infection of the incision without involvement of the device pocket is one exception to this dictum.[16,55,58,62]

A study examining 123 patients with PPM or ICD infections, found that only 1 out of 117 (1%) patients who had complete device extraction experienced relapsed infection, whereas 3 out of 6 (50%) patients who did not have complete device removal relapsed during a mean follow-up of 56 weeks (range 1 week–194 weeks).[55] The single patient who relapsed with complete device extraction had new hardware placed in the old pocket. Another series of 39 patients with CIED infection found no relapses among the patients with complete device extraction, but 67% of patients with partial device removal or conservative therapy developed recurrent infection.[66] These findings are mirrored by another large study that found a low incidence of relapsed infection with complete device extraction (5 out of 142; 3.5%). Notably, most relapses occurred in patients with partial hardware removal.[16] As with other device-associated infections, it is thought that tight grouping of bacteria with polysaccharide cell-to-cell adhesion molecules, referred to as biofilm, contributes to high recurrence rates in the absence of device removal. The extracellular matrix forming the biofilm may impede access to the host defenses and limit the efficacy of antimicrobials.[69]

S Aureus Bacteremia

The management of S aureus bacteremia (SAB) among patients with a CIED who do not have clinical evidence of generator-site infection, lead vegetation, or valve vegetation remains challenging. Prospective studies suggest the incidence of CIED infection may be as high as 45% in patients with SAB,[57] and a portion of these patients may not have localizing signs or symptoms. However, universal extraction of CIED devices in all patients with SAB is also not appropriate. Certain clinical scenarios increase the probability of CIED infection and should prompt clinicians to strongly consider device extraction. These scenarios include SAB without another identified source,[57,62] recurrent SAB,[57,62,68,70] persistent bacteremia ($\geq$24 hours),[62,68] presence of a prosthetic valve,[62,71] presence of an ICD,[71] and bacteremia within 3 months of device placement.[57,62]

An investigation of 23 patients with recurrent SAB found that recurrence that occurred after appropriate antimicrobial therapy frequently represented an occult infection of an indwelling foreign body (P<.001).[70] A prospective study of 33 patients with PPMs or ICDs and SAB found that 70% of patients had either confirmed (45.4%) or possible (24.6%) CIED infections.[57] Most patients (75%) with early SAB (<1 year after device implantation) had confirmed CIED infection. In contrast, 28.5% of patients with SAB at or greater than 1 year after device implantation had confirmed CIED infection and 43% had possible CIED infection. In early SAB, the CIED was the primary source of bacteremia in 67% of patients, whereas 33% of patients developed hematogenous seeding from a distant or unknown primary source. In contrast, all the patients with late SAB developed hematogenous seeding of their device from a distant or unknown primary source of S aureus infection. In 17% of patients who underwent echocardiography, neither lead wire vegetation nor valvular vegetation was identified despite S aureus being isolated from the generator pocket. In addition, local signs of device involvement were seen in only 40% of patients. Based on these findings, the investigators concluded that identifying CIED infection in patients with SAB might be difficult because clinical signs of pocket infection may not always be evident and TEE may not exclude infection of the generator pocket. In addition, the investigators advocated that most patients with a CIED who develop SAB should undergo device extraction. Circumstances in which device extraction should strongly be considered include clinical or echocardiographic evidence of CIED infection, recurrent SAB, or SAB without an identifiable source—even when clinical or echocardiographic evidence of CIED infection is absent.

Another retrospective investigation by Uslan and colleagues[71] reported that 35.5% (22 out of 62 patients) of patients with SAB and a CIED had a device infection. In this study, device-related endocarditis represented most CIED infections (55%) followed by generator pocket infection (31.7%). Risk factors for device-related endocarditis among patients without generator pocket infection included presence of ICD (OR 13.3; CI 2.1–84.9) and presence of a prosthetic valve (OR 6.8; CI 1.1–43.4). The reasons for an increased rate of infection in ICD recipients compared with PPM recipients was not clear, but, in this population, more ICD recipients were anticoagulated, had congestive heart failure, or underwent multiple device procedures. The increased complexity of ICD leads (more irregular contours and texture compared with PPM leads), may also contribute to the increased risk of infection. Similar to findings by Chamis and colleagues,[57] two patients did not have vegetation on TEE but later met criteria for CIED- associated endocarditis when the extracted lead tip culture was positive for S aureus.

A recent scientific statement from the AHA recommended device extraction in the setting of SAB without an identifiable source.[62] This recommendation contrasts with the usual management of a CIED in the setting of gram-negative bacteremia. A study examining 49 patients with a PPM or ICD and gram-negative bacteremia reported that only 6% of patients had either definite or possible CIED infection. No patients seemed to have secondary hematogenous seeding of the system.[72] Thus, device extraction in the setting of gram-negative bacteremia is not recommended without clinical or echocardiographic evidence of CIED infection unless bacteremia is persistent or relapses without another defined focus of infection.[62]

Explantation

Historically, surgical lead removal with a thoracotomy was considered in patients with vegetation diameters less than 10 mm or with retained hardware after failed attempts with percutaneous lead removal.[58,73–75] The preference for surgical approach among patients with larger vegetations was based in large part on previous investigations of patients with infective endocarditis (valve infections) in which vegetation diameters greater than 10 mm were associated with a significantly higher incidence of embolic events than vegetation diameters less than 10 mm.[76] Although some studies support a relationship between vegetation size and risk of pulmonary embolus, other studies have not found such a correlation.[58]

Recently, multiple centers have reported successful experiences with percutaneous lead removal in the setting of large lead-associated vegetation.[16,56,77–79] One study found that 96% (182 out of 189) of patients with CIED infection underwent complete device extraction at the time of initial presentation and 90% of the device removals were performed by percutaneous lead extraction.[16] Among the patients who had percutaneous lead extraction, the diameter of the lead-associated vegetations or valvular vegetations ranged from 0.3 to 7.0 cm in longest dimension, but none of these patients developed clinically apparent pulmonary embolus. Another study found that transvenous pacemaker lead removal was safe among patients with vegetations larger than 1 cm.[78] Embolism of the vegetation into the pulmonary circulation did occur in a few patients, but no clinical complications resulted. In this study, most patients with vegetations larger than 2 cm diameter underwent open heart surgery because of concern for embolism that could obstruct the main stem of the pulmonary artery. However, several patients with vegetations larger than 2 cm successfully underwent transvenous lead removal.

A recent update on the management on CIED infections and a poll of an expert panel advocated that percutaneous removal could be performed safely at high-volume centers when lead vegetations are smaller than 2 cm.[62,80] With vegetations larger than 2 cm there are limited data on the appropriateness of percutaneous versus surgical removal. The decision regarding approach should be individualized.[62]

Complications from percutaneous lead extraction may occur, so these procedures should only be performed at facilities where immediate assistance by cardiac surgery is available. In a larger series of patients that underwent percutaneous lead extraction, 11% of patients developed complications necessitating surgical intervention.[16] Specific complications included damage to the tricuspid valve, subclavian vein laceration, hemothorax, pocket hematoma, and fracture of lead tip. Analysis of a large database of 3540 CIED lead extractions from 2338 patients in the mid-1990s reported that the risk of complication increased with the number of leads removed, less experienced physicians, and female patients.[81] Referral to high-volume centers is strongly advised because the associated risks of lead extraction, in large measure, depends on the experience of the extraction physician and his or her team.[82,83]

Antimicrobial Treatment

Robust evidence for the optimal duration of antimicrobial treatment for different types of CIED infections is limited. A retrospective analysis of 189 patients with CIED infections as well as a recent scientific statement from the AHA, provide guidance on the duration of antimicrobial therapy for different types of CIED infections (**Fig. 2**A).[16,62] Some important findings by Sohail and colleagues[16] provide part of the basis for the proposed algorithm. For the cohort of 189 patients, the observed cure rate was 96% with both complete device removal and antimicrobial therapy. Pocket infections were treated with 10 to 14 days of antimicrobials, patients with bacteremia were treated with 4 weeks of antimicrobials, and patients with right-sided endocarditis were treated with 4 weeks of antimicrobials. Patients with CNS infection had a significantly shorter treatment course compared with patients with S aureus CIED infection (14 days vs 28 days; $P<.001$).

The proposed algorithm (see **Fig. 2**A) recommends a 7 to 10 day course of antimicrobials from the day of device explantation for generator or lead erosion without

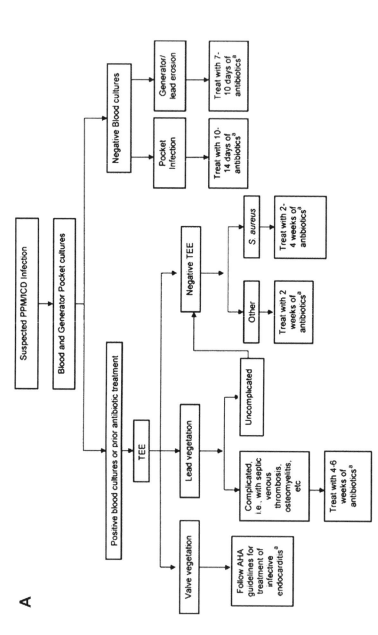

Fig. 2. (A) Approach to antimicrobial treatment of adults with CIED infection. This algorithm applies only to the patients with complete device explantation. [a]Duration of antibiotics should be counted from the day of device explantation. (B) Algorithm for reimplantation of new device in patients with CIED infection. ([Panel A] Reprinted from Sohail M, Uslan D, Khan A, et al. Management and outcome of permanent pacemaker and implantable cardioverter-defibrillator infections. J Am Coll Cardiol 2007;49(18):1851–9; with permission.)

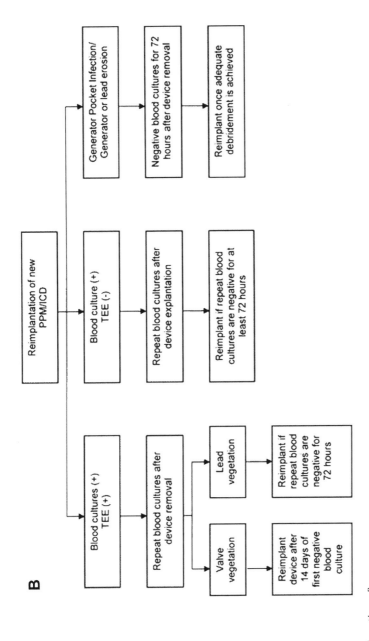

Fig. 2. (continued)

bacteremia. Pocket infections without bacteremia may be treated with 10 to 14 days of antimicrobials from the day of device explantation. When a generator pocket infection is complicated by bacteremia and a TEE does not show a lead or valvular vegetation, then two weeks of parenteral antimicrobials should be sufficient in most circumstances. Clinicians should repeat blood cultures after device explantation in patients with bacteremia, and a minimum of 4 weeks of antimicrobials should be administered in patients with sustained bacteremia after CIED removal.[16] A longer duration of therapy is also appropriate in patients with complications such as osteomyelitis, deep abscess, septic arthritis, or septic thrombophlebitis. Based on recent Infectious Disease Society of America guidelines addressing the management of methicillin resistant *S aureus* (MRSA) infection, patients with SAB in the setting of a CIED infection are classified as complicated SAB and they should receive 4 to 6 weeks of antimicrobial therapy.[84] This recommendation differs from the 2 to 4 week duration of antimicrobial therapy for CIED infection and SAB (without endocarditis) recommended by the AHA.[62]

For patients with device-related valvular vegetations, the choice and duration of antimicrobial therapy is pathogen specific and AHA guidelines should be followed for treatment of infective endocarditis.[59] In the setting of MRSA native valve infective endocarditis, recent clinical guidelines for treatment of MRSA infections recommend vancomycin or daptomycin for 6 weeks.[84] The routine addition of rifampin or gentamicin is not recommended for treatment of MRSA native valve infective endocarditis. The duration of antimicrobials for lead vegetations without additional complications requires clarification.[26,85] A shorter duration of therapy (2 weeks) can be considered in patients without secondary complications from the lead vegetation and when the pathogen is not *S aureus*.

Timing of Device Replacement

After extraction of an infected CIED, all patients should be assessed for whether a CIED is still necessary (see **Fig. 2B**). Owing to a variety of factors, such as improvement in clinical status or initial lack of appropriate indication, one-third to one-half of patients may not require a new CIED implantation.[16,55,56] Patients who are PPM dependent may benefit from active-fixation (screw-in) leads attached to the externalized infected generators as a bridge until PPM implantation is deemed appropriate. This approach is associated with less dislodgement than the traditional temporary pacemaker wires and fosters early patient ambulation.[86] There is very limited experience with simultaneous, contralateral CIED replacement; therefore, this approach is not recommended for routine use.[87]

To date, there are no prospective trials examining the risk of recurrent infection based on timing of CIED replacement and variability in practices exist. In a recent series of 39 patients with CIED infection, 54% underwent reimplantation a median of 28 days (1–74 days) after extraction without further relapse of infection.[66] Another study examining the management of 189 patient with CIED infection, found the median time to reimplantation was significantly longer in patients with bacteremia compared with those without bacteremia (13 days vs 7 days; $P<.0001$).[16] Five percent of patients experienced a relapse of infection; most underwent only partial hardware removal. For patients with generator erosion or lead erosion, the median time from explantation to reimplantation was only 3 days and none of the patients experienced infection relapse. A low rate of infection relapse (4%) with earlier reimplantation was also reported in a series of a 123 patients with CIED infection.[55] The median time to reimplantation of a new device was 5 days (0–68 days) and 7 out of 13 underwent reimplantation a median of 7 days after extraction. Often, clinicians believe that the presence of vegetation might increase the risk of relapse and that reimplantation should be delayed. However, a recent series of 100 patients with intracardiac vegetations reported a median time to replacement of 7 days; none of the patients who received a new CIED experienced a relapse of infection.[56]

A recent scientific statement from the AHA provides guidance on the appropriate timing of device replacement.[62] In the setting of bacteremia, the timing of new CIED implantation depends on clearance of bacteremia after device extraction and presence of valvular vegetations. For patients with valvular vegetations and bacteremia, reimplantation of a CIED device can be performed 14 days from the time of the first negative blood culture after device extraction. Patients who have a lead vegetation or bacteremia without device-associated endocarditis (ie, no valvular vegetation) can safely undergo implantation of a new CIED device when blood cultures drawn after device extraction are negative for 72 hours. In the setting of a generator pocket infection, generator erosion, or lead erosion, implantation of a new CIED can be performed when blood cultures are negative for 72 hours, provided there has been adequate debridement of the generator pocket. The importance of implantation on the contralateral side has been emphasized by multiple studies and is recommended in the AHA guidelines.[16,55,56] When implantation on the contralateral side is not possible, a transvenous lead can be tunneled to a device placed subcutaneously in the abdomen, or an epicardial system may be implanted.[62]

PREVENTION

Multiple studies have demonstrated that antimicrobial prophylaxis reduces the risk of CIED infection.[2,16,18,20,22] A meta-analysis of seven, small, randomized clinical trials examining the impact of systemic antimicrobial prophylaxis on the risk of PPM infection found a consistent protective effect of prophylaxis (OR 0.256; 95% CI: 0.10–0.656).[20] One major limitation of this meta-analysis was the variability in antimicrobial choice and duration of use among the studies. A recent randomized, double-blinded, placebo-controlled trial that included 1000 patients undergoing primary CIED implantation or generator replacement examined the efficacy of cefazolin prophylaxis during a 6 month follow-up period.[22] A single, one-gram dose of cefazolin was administered immediately before the procedure without weight-based dose adjustment or redosing during longer procedures. After 649 patients were enrolled, the patient safety committee interrupted the study because CIED infection occurred in 0.63% of patients receiving cefazolin and 3.28% of patients receiving placebo (relative risk 0.19; P = .016). Multivariable analysis identified antimicrobial nonuse and postoperative hematoma as independent predictors of infection. Future studies should address weight-based dosing recommendations and redosing intervals in longer procedures.[88,89]

The recent scientific statement by the AHA addressing the management of CIED infections recommends prophylaxis with an agent that has in vitro activity against staphylococci.[62] When cefazolin is used, it should be administered within 1 hour before incision and, if vancomycin is used, it should be administered intravenously within 2 hours of incision. Antimicrobial prophylaxis in the postoperative period is currently not recommended because of lack of supporting evidence and the potential risk of adverse drug effects or the development of antimicrobial resistance.

Recently, a case series evaluating an antibacterial envelope implanted in the generator pocket with the CIED was reported.[90] The envelope is a polymer mesh that releases rifampin and minocycline after implantation. Nearly half the patients (49%) in this study had at least three established risk factors for development of CIED infection, but there was a low rate of infection (<0.50%). Unfortunately, neither this nor other studies have included a control group. Prospective randomized trials demonstrating clinical efficacy and cost-effectiveness are needed before this approach can be recommended broadly. Nonetheless, future studies evaluating interventions that target high-risk patients are essential.

SUMMARY

CIED infections are an increasing problem associated with high morbidity and mortality. Major risk factors for CIED infection include renal insufficiency, presence of indwelling catheters, diabetes mellitus, and corticosteroid use. *Staphylococcus* spp are the most common pathogen, whereas gram-negative bacteria are rarely implicated. Blood cultures, generator pocket tissue cultures, lead tip cultures, and echocardiography are key aspects of the diagnostic work-up for suspected CIED infection. Complete removal of all hardware is strongly recommended, along with adjunctive antimicrobial therapy, unless the patient is at extremely high risk of periprocedural complications or has limited life expectancy. In such cases, chronic suppressive antimicrobial treatment may be preferred. Most studies examining the management of CIED infections are small and nonrandomized. Larger, multicenter, prospective studies are needed to better define optimal management strategies. Additionally, major emphasis should be placed on prevention of this often devastating complication.

REFERENCES

1. Uslan DZ, Sohail MR, St. Sauver JL, et al. Permanent pacemaker and implantable cardioverter defibrillator infection: a population-based study. Arch Intern Med 2007;167(7):669–75.
2. Klug D, Balde M, Pavin D, et al. Risk factors related to infections of implanted pacemakers and cardioverter-defibrillators: results of a large prospective study. Circulation 2007;116(12):1349–55.
3. Gregoratos G, Abrams J, Epstein AE, et al. ACC/AHA/NASPE 2002 guideline update for implantation of cardiac pacemakers and antiarrhythmia devices: summary article: a report of the American College of Cardiology/American Heart Association Task Force on Practice Guidelines (ACC/AHA/NASPE Committee to Update the 1998 Pacemaker Guidelines). Circulation 2002;106(16):2145–61.
4. Epstein AE, DiMarco JP, Ellenbogen KA, et al. ACC/AHA/HRS 2008 guidelines for device-based therapy of cardiac rhythm abnormalities: a report of the American College of Cardiology/American Heart Association Task Force on Practice Guidelines (Writing Committee to Revise the ACC/AHA/NASPE 2002 Guideline Update for Implantation of Cardiac Pacemakers and Antiarrhythmia Devices): developed in collaboration with the American Association for Thoracic Surgery and Society of Thoracic Surgeons. Circulation 2008;117(21):e350–408.
5. Proclemer A, Ghidina M, Cicuttini G, et al. Impact of the main implantable cardioverter-defibrillator trials for primary and secondary prevention in Italy: a survey of the national activity during the years 2001–2004. Pacing Clin Electrophysiol 2006;29:S20–8.
6. Uslan DZ, Tleyjeh IM, Baddour LM, et al. Temporal trends in permanent pacemaker implantation: a population-based study. Am Heart J 2008;155(5):896–903.
7. Zhan C, Baine WB, Sedrakyan A, et al. Cardiac device implantation in the United States from 1997 through 2004: a population-based analysis. J Gen Intern Med 2008;23(Suppl 1):13–9.

8. Voigt A, Shalaby A, Saba S. Rising rates of cardiac rhythm management device infections in the United States: 1996 through 2003. J Am Coll Cardiol 2006;48(3): 590–1.
9. Mirowski M, Reid PR, Mower MM, et al. Termination of malignant ventricular arrhythmias with an implanted automatic defibrillator in human beings. N Engl J Med 1980;303(6):322–4.
10. Lai KK, Fontecchio SA. Infections associated with implantable cardioverter defibrillators placed transvenously and via thoracotomies: epidemiology, infection control, and management. Clin Infect Dis 1998;27(2):265–9.
11. Mela T, McGovern BA, Garan H, et al. Long-term infection rates associated with the pectoral versus abdominal approach to cardioverter- defibrillator implants. Am J Cardiol 2001;88(7):750–3.
12. Gold MR, Peters RW, Johnson JW, et al. Complications associated with pectoral cardioverter-defibrillator implantation: comparison of subcutaneous and submuscular approaches. J Am Coll Cardiol 1996;28(5):1278–82.
13. Cabell CH, Heidenreich PA, Chu VH, et al. Increasing rates of cardiac device infections among Medicare beneficiaries: 1990-1999. Am Heart J 2004;147(4): 582–6.
14. Lin G, Meverden R, Hodge D, et al. Age and gender trends in implantable cardioverter defibrillator utilization: a population based study. J Interv Card Electrophysiol 2008;22(1):65–70.
15. Bloom H, Heeke B, Leon A, et al. Renal insufficiency and the risk of infection from pacemaker or defibrillator surgery. Pacing Clin Electrophysiol 2006;29(2):142–5.
16. Sohail MR, Uslan D, Khan AH, et al. Management and outcome of permanent pacemaker and implantable cardioverter-defibrillator infections. J Am Coll Cardiol 2007;49(18):1851–9.
17. Sohail MR, Hussain S, Le KY, et al. Risk factors associated with early- versus late-onset implantable cardioverter-defibrillator infections. J Interv Card Electrophysiol 2011;31(2):171–83, 1–13.
18. Cengiz M, Okutucu S, Ascioglu S, et al. Permanent pacemaker and implantable cardioverter defibrillator infections: seven years of diagnostic and therapeutic experience of a single center. Clin Cardiol 2010;33(7):406–11.
19. Turakhia MP, Varosy PD, Lee K, et al. Impact of renal function on survival in patients with implantable cardioverter-defibrillators. Pacing Clin Electrophysiol 2007;30(3):377–84.
20. Da Costa A, Kirkorian G, Cucherat M, et al. Antibiotic prophylaxis for permanent pacemaker implantation: a meta-analysis. Circulation 1998;97(18):1796–801.
21. Nery PB, Fernandes R, Nair GM, et al. Device-related infection among patients with pacemakers and implantable defibrillators: incidence, risk factors, and consequences. J Cardiovasc Electrophysiol 2010;21(7):786–90.
22. de Oliveira JC, Martinelli M, Nishioka SA, et al. Efficacy of antibiotic prophylaxis before the implantation of pacemakers and cardioverter-defibrillators. Circ Arrhythm Electrophysiol 2009;2(1):29–34.
23. Aggarwal RK, Connelly DT, Ray SG, et al. Early complications of permanent pacemaker implantation: no difference between dual and single chamber systems. Br Heart J 1995;73(6):571–5.
24. Chauhan A, Grace AA, Newell SA, et al. Early complications after dual chamber versus single chamber pacemaker implantation. Pacing Clin Electrophysiol 1994;17(11 Pt 2):2012–5.
25. Poole J, Gleva M, Mela T, et al. Complication rates associated with pacemaker or implantable cardioverter-defibrillator generator replacements and upgrade

procedures: results from the REPLACE registry. Circulation 2010;122(16): 1553–61.

26. Sohail MR, Uslan DZ, Khan AH, et al. Infective endocarditis complicating permanent pacemaker and implantable cardioverter-defibrillator infection. Mayo Clin Proc 2008;83(1):46–53.

27. Massoure PL, Reuter S, Lafitte S, et al. Pacemaker endocarditis: clinical features and management of 60 consecutive cases. Pacing Clin Electrophysiol 2007; 30(1):12–9.

28. Rundstrom H, Kennergren C, Andersson R, et al. Pacemaker endocarditis during 18 years in Goteborg. Scand J Infect Dis 2004;36(9):674–9.

29. Takigawa M, Noda T, Kurita T, et al. Extremely late pacemaker-infective endocarditis due to Stenotrophomonas maltophilia. Cardiology 2008;110(4):226–9.

30. Marull JM, De Benedetti ME. Automatic implantable cardioverter defibrillator pocket infection due to *Providencia rettgeri*: a case report. Cases J 2009;2:8607.

31. Ahn Y, Kim NH, Shin DH, et al. Pacemaker lead endocarditis caused by *Achromobacter xylosoxidans*. J Korean Med Sci 2004;19(2):291–3.

32. Duan X, Ling F, Zhou L, et al. Pacemaker generator pocket infection due to *Burkholderia cepacia*. J Hosp Infect 2007;67(4):392–3.

33. Metallidis S, Chrysanthidis T, Kazakos E, et al. A fatal case of pacemaker lead endocarditis caused by Mucor spp. Int J Infect Dis 2008;12(6):e151–2.

34. Cook RJ, Orszulak TA, Nkomo VT, et al. Aspergillus infection of implantable cardioverter-defibrillator. Mayo Clin Proc 2004;79(4):549–52.

35. Dunn CJ, Ruder M, Deresinski SC. *Aspergillus fumigatus* infection of an automatic internal cardiac defibrillator. Pacing Clin Electrophysiol 1996;19(12 Pt 1):2156–7.

36. Izquierdo R, Llorente C, Mayo J, et al. Pacemaker infection due to Aspergillus: report of two cases and literature review. Clin Cardiol 2005;28(1):36–8.

37. Marchena Yglesias PJ, Rodriguez JA, Garcia GA, et al. Pacemaker lead infection caused by *Aspergillus fumigatus*. Eur J Intern Med 2006;17(3):209–10.

38. Heitmann L, Cometta A, Hurni M, et al. Right-sided pacemaker-related endocarditis due to *Acremonium* species. Clin Infect Dis 1997;25(1):158–60.

39. Kouvousis N, Lazaros G, Christoforatou E, et al. Pacemaker pocket infection due to *Acremonium* species. Pacing Clin Electrophysiol 2002;25(3):378–9.

40. Tascini C, Bongiorni MG, Leonildi A, et al. Pacemaker endocarditis with pulmonary cavitary lesion due to *Scedosporium prolificans*. J Chemother 2006;18(6):667–9.

41. Sarvat B, Sarria JC. Implantable cardioverter-defibrillator infection due to *Scedosporium apiospermum*. J Infect 2007;55(4):e109–13.

42. Laurini JA, Carter JE, Kahn AG. Tricuspid valve and pacemaker endocarditis due to *Pseudallescheria boydii* (*Scedosporium apiospermum*). South Med J 2009;102(5):515–7.

43. Foo H, Ooi SY, Giles R, et al. *Scedosporium apiospermum* pacemaker endocarditis. Int J Cardiol 2009;131(2):e81–2.

44. Marchandin H, Battistella P, Calvet B, et al. Pacemaker surgical site infection caused by *Mycobacterium goodii*. J Med Microbiol 2009;58(Pt 4):517–20.

45. Chrissoheris MP, Kadakia H, Marieb M, et al. Pacemaker pocket infection due to *Mycobacterium goodii*: case report and review of the literature. Conn Med 2008; 72(2):75–7.

46. Toda H, Sato K, Iimori M, et al. A case of *Mycobacterium goodii* infection wifh isolation from blood and a pacemaker lead. Kansenshogaku Zasshi 2006; 80(3):262–6 [in Japanese].

47. Tam WO, Yew WW, Yam WC, et al. Pacemaker infections due to rapidly growing mycobacteria: further experience. Int J Tuberc Lung Dis 2007;11(1):118.

48. Giannella M, Valerio M, Franco JA, et al. Pacemaker infection due to *Mycobacterium fortuitum*: the role of universal 16S rRNA gene PCR and sequencing. Diagn Microbiol Infect Dis 2007;57(3):337–9.
49. Al Soub H, Al Maslamani M, Al Khuwaiter J, et al. Myocardial abscess and bacteremia complicating *Mycobacterium fortuitum* pacemaker infection: case report and review of the literature. Pediatr Infect Dis J 2009;28(11):1032–4.
50. Cutay AM, Horowitz HW, Pooley RW, et al. Infection of epicardial pacemaker wires due to *Mycobacterium abscessus*. Clin Infect Dis 1998;26(2):520–1.
51. Kessler AT, Kourtis AP. *Mycobacterium abscessus* as a cause of pacemaker infection. Med Sci Monit 2004;10(10):CS60–2.
52. Kestler M, Reves R, Belknap R. Pacemaker wire infection with *Mycobacterium tuberculosis*: a case report and literature review. Int J Tuberc Lung Dis 2009; 13(2):272–4.
53. Luckie M, Zaidi A, Woodhead M, et al. *Mycobacterium tuberculosis* causing infection of an implantable biventricular defibrillator. Indian J Tuberc 2010;57(4):213–5.
54. Hellwig T, Ou P, Offredo C, et al. Unusual chronic pacemaker infection by *Mycobacterium tuberculosis* in a pediatric patient. J Thorac Cardiovasc Surg 2005; 130(3):937–8.
55. Chua JD, Wilkoff BL, Lee I, et al. Diagnosis and management of infections involving implantable electrophysiologic cardiac devices. Ann Intern Med 2000;133(8):604–8.
56. Grammes J, Schulze C, Al-Bataineh M, et al. Percutaneous pacemaker and implantable cardioverter-defibrillator lead extraction in 100 patients with intracardiac vegetations defined by transesophageal echocardiogram. J Am Coll Cardiol 2010;55(9):886–94.
57. Chamis AL, Peterson GE, Cabell CH, et al. *Staphylococcus aureus* bacteremia in patients with permanent pacemakers or implantable cardioverter-defibrillators. Circulation 2001;104(9):1029–33.
58. Klug D, Lacroix D, Savoye C, et al. Systemic infection related to endocarditis on pacemaker leads: clinical presentation and management. Circulation 1997; 95(8):2098–107.
59. Baddour LM, Wilson WR, Bayer AS, et al. Infective endocarditis: diagnosis, antimicrobial therapy, and management of complications: a statement for healthcare professionals from the Committee on Rheumatic Fever, Endocarditis, and Kawasaki Disease, Council on Cardiovascular Disease in the Young, and the Councils on Clinical Cardiology, Stroke, and Cardiovascular Surgery and Anesthesia, American Heart Association: Endorsed by the Infectious Diseases Society of America. Circulation 2005;111(23):e394–434.
60. del Río A, Anguera I, Miró JM, et al. Surgical treatment of pacemaker and defibrillator lead endocarditis: the impact of electrode lead extraction on outcome. Chest 2003;124(4):1451–9.
61. Klug D, Wallet F, Lacroix D, et al. Local symptoms at the site of pacemaker implantation indicate latent systemic infection. Heart 2004;90(8):882–6.
62. Baddour LM, Epstein AE, Erickson CC, et al. Update on cardiovascular implantable electronic device infections and their management: a scientific statement from the American Heart Association. Circulation 2010;121(3):458–77.
63. Dy Chua J, Abdul-Karim A, Mawhorter S, et al. The role of swab and tissue culture in the diagnosis of implantable cardiac device infection. Pacing Clin Electrophysiol 2005;28(12):1276–81.
64. Downey BC, Juselius WE, Pandian NG, et al. Incidence and significance of pacemaker and implantable cardioverter-defibrillator lead masses discovered

during transesophageal echocardiography. Pacing Clin Electrophysiol 2011; 34(6):679–83.

65. Fowler VG, Li J, Corey GR, et al. Role of echocardiography in evaluation of patients with *Staphylococcus aureus* bacteremia: experience in 103 patients. J Am Coll Cardiol 1997;30(4):1072–8.

66. Margey R, McCann H, Blake G, et al. Contemporary management of and outcomes from cardiac device related infections. Europace 2010;12(1):64–70.

67. Cacoub P, Leprince P, Nataf P, et al. Pacemaker infective endocarditis. Am J Cardiol 1998;82(4):480–4.

68. Camus C, Leport C, Raffi F, et al. Sustained bacteremia in 26 patients with a permanent endocardial pacemaker: assessment of wire removal. Clin Infect Dis 1993;17(1):46–55.

69. Heilmann C, Gerke C, Perdreau-Remington F, et al. Characterization of Tn917 insertion mutants of *Staphylococcus epidermidis* affected in biofilm formation. Infect Immun 1996;64(1):277–82.

70. Fowler VG, Kong LK, Corey GR, et al. Recurrent *Staphylococcus aureus* bacteremia: pulsed-field gel electrophoresis findings in 29 patients. J Infect Dis 1999; 179(5):1157–61.

71. Uslan DZ, Dowsley TF, Sohail MR, et al. Cardiovascular implantable electronic device infection in patients with *Staphylococcus aureus* bacteremia. Pacing Clin Electrophysiol 2010;33(4):407–13.

72. Uslan DZ, Sohail MR, Friedman PA, et al. Frequency of permanent pacemaker or implantable cardioverter-defibrillator infection in patients with gram-negative bacteremia. Clin Infect Dis 2006;43(6):731–6.

73. Frame R, Brodman RF, Furman S, et al. Surgical removal of infected transvenous pacemaker leads. Pacing Clin Electrophysiol 1993;16(12):2343–8.

74. Miralles A, Moncada V, Chevez H, et al. Pacemaker endocarditis: approach for lead extraction in endocarditis with large vegetations. Ann Thorac Surg 2001; 72(6):2130–2.

75. Camboni D, Wollmann C, Lher A, et al. Explantation of implantable defibrillator leads using open heart surgery or percutaneous techniques. Ann Thorac Surg 2008;85(1):50–5.

76. Mugge A, Daniel WG, Frank G, et al. Echocardiography in infective endocarditis: reassessment of prognostic implications of vegetation size determined by the trans-thoracic and the transesophageal approach. J Am Coll Cardiol 1989;14(3):631–8.

77. Nguyen KT, Neese P, Kessler DJ. Successful laser-assisted percutaneous extraction of four pacemaker leads associated with large vegetations. Pacing Clin Electrophysiol 2000;23(8):1260–2.

78. Ruttmann E, Hangler HB, Kilo J, et al. Transvenous pacemaker lead removal is safe and effective even in large vegetations: an analysis of 53 cases of pacemaker lead endocarditis. Pacing Clin Electrophysiol 2006;29(3):231–6.

79. Calton R, Cameron D, Cusimano RJ, et al. Successful laser-assisted removal of an infected ICD lead with a large vegetation. Pacing Clin Electrophysiol 2006; 29(8):910–3.

80. Field ME, Jones SO, Epstein LM. How to select patients for lead extraction. Heart Rhythm 2007;4(7):978–85.

81. Byrd CL, Wilkoff BL, Love CJ, et al. Intravascular extraction of problematic or infected permanent pacemaker leads: 1994-1996. U.S. Extraction Database, MED Institute. Pacing Clin Electrophysiol 1999;22(9):1348–57.

82. Wilkoff BL, Love CJ, Byrd CL, et al. Transvenous lead extraction: Heart Rhythm Society expert consensus on facilities, training, indications, and patient

management: this document was endorsed by the American Heart Association (AHA). Heart Rhythm 2009;6(7):1085–104.

83. Ghosh N, Yee R, Klein GJ, et al. Laser lead extraction: is there a learning curve? Pacing Clin Electrophysiol 2005;28(3):180–4.

84. Liu C, Bayer A, Cosgrove SE, et al. Clinical practice guidelines by the infectious Diseases Society of America for the treatment of methicillin-resistant *Staphylococcus aureus* infections in adults and children. Clin Infect Dis 2011;52(3): e18–55.

85. Dumont E, Camus C, Victor F, et al. Suspected pacemaker or defibrillator transvenous lead infection. Eur Heart J 2003;24(19):1779–87.

86. Braun MU, Rauwolf T, Bock M, et al. Percutaneous lead implantation connected to an external device in stimulation-dependent patients with systemic infection—a prospective and controlled study. Pacing Clin Electrophysiol 2006; 29(8):875–9.

87. Nandyala R, Parsonnet V. One stage side-to-side replacement of infected pulse generators and leads. Pacing Clin Electrophysiol 2006;29(4):393–6.

88. Bratzler DW, Hunt DR. The surgical infection prevention and surgical care improvement projects: national initiatives to improve outcomes for patients having surgery. Clin Infect Dis 2006;43(3):322–30.

89. Bratzler DW, Houck PM. Antimicrobial prophylaxis for surgery: an advisory statement from the National Surgical Infection Prevention Project. Am J Surg 2005;189(4):395–404.

90. Bloom HL, Constantin L, Dan D, et al. Implantation success and infection in cardiovascular implantable electronic device procedures utilizing an antibacterial envelope. Pacing Clin Electrophysiol 2011;34(2):133–42.

91. Celard M, Vandenesch F, Darbas H, et al. Pacemaker infection caused by *Staphylococcus schleiferi*, a member of the human preaxillary flora: four case reports. Clin Infect Dis 1997;24(5):1014–5.

92. Dhand A, Ross JJ. Implantable cardioverter-defibrillator infection due to *Brucella melitensis*: case report and review of brucellosis of cardiac devices. Clin Infect Dis 2007;44(4):e37–9.

93. de la Fuente A, Sanchez JR, Uriz J, et al. Infection of a pacemaker by *Brucella melitensis*. Tex Heart Inst J 1997;24(2):129–30.

94. Francia E, Domingo P, Sambeat MA, et al. Pacemaker infection by *Brucella melitensis*: a rare cause of relapsing brucellosis. Arch Intern Med 2000;160(21): 3327–8.

95. Kimmel M, Kuhlmann U, Alscher DM. Pacemaker infection with propionibacterium and a nephritic sediment. Clin Nephrol 2008;69(2):127–9.

96. Abusin S, Bhimaraj A, Khadra S. Bacillus Cereus Endocarditis in a permanent pacemaker: a case report. Cases J 2008;1(1):95.

97. Boell K, Gotoff R, Foltzer M, et al. Implantable defibrillator pocket infection and bacteremia caused by *Nocardia nova* complex isolate. J Clin Microbiol 2003; 41(11):5325–6.

98. Ahmar W, Johnson D, Richards M, et al. Campylobacter fetus infection of an internal cardioverter defibrillator. Pacing Clin Electrophysiol 2008;31(2):258–9.

99. Cikes M, Mookadam M, Asirvatham SJ, et al. Pseudomonas infection of implantable cardioverter-defibrillator generator and leads as a complication of gastrostomy. Int J Infect Dis 2007;11(3):281–2.

100. Chacko ST, Chandy ST, Abraham OC, et al. Pacemaker endocarditis caused by *Pseudomonas aeruginosa* treated successfully. J Assoc Physicians India 2003; 51:1021–2.

101. Cohen TJ, Pons VG, Schwartz J, et al. *Candida albicans* pacemaker site infection. Pacing Clin Electrophysiol 1991;14(2 Pt 1):146–8.
102. Kurup A, Janardhan MN, Seng TY. *Candida tropicalis* pacemaker endocarditis. J Infect 2000;41(3):275–6.
103. Amin M, Gross J, Andrews C, et al. Pacemaker infection with *Mycobacterium avium* complex. Pacing Clin Electrophysiol 1991;14(2 Pt 1):152–4.
104. Katona P, Wiener I, Saxena N. *Mycobacterium avium-intracellulare* infection of an automatic implantable cardioverter defibrillator. Am Heart J 1992;124(5):1380–1.

Left Ventricular Assist Device– Associated Infections

Sophia Califano, MD[a], Francis D. Pagani, MD, PhD[b],
Preeti N. Malani, MD, MSJ[c],*

KEYWORDS

- Left ventricular assist devices • Driveline infection
- Heart transplantation

Heart failure remains a major contributor to morbidity and mortality throughout the world. Although cardiac transplantation is a potentially lifesaving treatment for patients with end-stage disease, it relies on a limited number of donors, so many patients do not survive until an appropriate donor organ becomes available. In addition, many patients with heart failure are not candidates for transplantation because of significant comorbidities.

The left ventricular assist device (LVAD) is a mechanical pump that supplements or replaces the function of a damaged left ventricle to maintain appropriate blood flow among patients with end-stage heart failure. Use of LVADs was initially approved for use as a bridge to transplant, with the aim of increasing patient survival until an appropriate organ became available; however, indications have since expanded to include permanent implantation as an alternative to heart transplantation.

LVAD placement has been shown to be superior to maximal medical therapy in some patients, but its use continues to be associated with a high complication rate, most notably infection. The incidence of infection is between 18% and 59% of all implantations,[1-6] even causing death in a decreasing but significant percentage of patients. In this review, the authors provide an overview on the epidemiology of LVAD use and discuss associated infections, including risk factors, management, and prevention.

The authors have nothing to disclose. There was no outside support for this work.

[a] Department of Internal Medicine, University of Michigan, 1500 East Medical Center Drive, Ann Arbor, MI 48109, USA
[b] Adult Heart Transplantation, Center for Circulatory Support, University of Michigan, Ann Arbor, MI, USA
[c] Department of Internal Medicine, Divisions of Infectious Diseases and Geriatric Medicine, University of Michigan and Ann Arbor Veterans Affairs Ann Arbor Healthcare System, Geriatric Research Education and Clinical Center, 2215 Fuller Road, 111-I, 8th Floor, Ann Arbor, MI 48105, USA
* Corresponding author.
E-mail address: pmalani@umich.edu

Infect Dis Clin N Am 26 (2012) 77–87
doi:10.1016/j.idc.2011.09.008
0891-5520/12/$ – see front matter © 2012 Elsevier Inc. All rights reserved.

OVERVIEW OF LVADs

An estimated 5.7 million people in the United States are affected by heart failure, with 670,000 new cases per year[7] and an attributable cost of more than 39 billion dollars in 2010.[8] Current medical therapy remains grounded in the use of angiotensin-converting enzyme inhibitors, β-blockers, and diuretics, and although there have been some improvements in outcomes with aggressive medical therapy, these gains have been limited. Transplant remains a definitive treatment but relies on a relatively fixed number of donor organs.[9] Current estimates suggest that on any given day, there are approximately 3000 people in the United States who are on the transplant waiting list, and only about 2000 donor hearts become available each year.[10] The 2009 report of the Scientific Registry of Transplant Recipients on the state of heart transplantation noted an increase in both incidence and prevalence of heart failure, with a plateau in the number of transplants performed and the death of 1 patient on the waiting list for every 5 patients who received a heart transplant.[11]

The LVAD was first conceived as an implantable, durable, and transportable device to provide circulatory support for patients with end-stage heart failure in the ambulatory setting and has undergone a rapid evolution since its inception. Because most cases of severe heart failure originate on the stronger left side of the heart, LVADs are engineered to preferentially support the left ventricle, although the same ventricular assist device (VAD) technology has also been used for right ventricular and biventricular support. Extended use of these devices is uncommon and beyond the scope of this review. The modern-day LVAD pumps are fully implantable but do require uninterrupted connection to a portable, although often sizeable, external power source.

In 1994, the original HeartMate (Thoratec, Pleasanton, CA, USA) LVAD gained US Food and Drug Administration (FDA) approval for general use as bridge therapy for patients awaiting transplant. In 2001, the REMATCH (Randomized Evaluation of Mechanical Assistance for the Treatment of Congestive Heart Failure) trial demonstrated improved 1-year survival rate with LVAD placement compared with medical therapy alone, and, subsequently, the LVAD gained approval for use as destination therapy among patients ineligible for transplant.[12]

At present, multiple groups of patients may benefit from LVAD support. However, the major indications for extended support remain the bridge-to-transplant and destination therapy groups, with the latter group often including older adults or patients with severe pulmonary or end-stage renal disease. In addition to supporting circulation, there is evidence that VAD placement can lead to other cardiac benefits, such as improved contractility, reduction of hypertrophy and fibrosis, and reversal of chamber enlargement.[13–17]

Most LVADs are surgically implanted via median sternotomy, with pump placement primarily in the intra-abdominal or preperitoneal space, with a percutaneous driveline leading to an external power source/air vent. Some devices used for short-term support are now being placed percutaneously. VAD designs generally fall into 2 major categories: pulsatile and continuous flow devices.

The first-generation devices were designed to mimic nature by providing pulsatile circulation. This concept was based on the belief that nonpulsatile flow delivered inadequate perfusion to distal vasculature, leading to weakening of muscle walls of major arteries. Engineering such pulsatile flow proved difficult and required many moving parts, including a diaphragm to hold and eject blood, valves to maintain directionality, and an air vent and conduit for cooling of the working parts. These requirements resulted in limitations in durability and size. With many movable parts, these devices begin to wear out during the first 2 years of use, and the large size necessitates placement in the preperitoneal space or intraperitoneal space.

The second-generation continuous flow devices are smaller than their first-generation counterparts and have fewer moving parts. These devices generally consist of inflow and outflow pumps and a rotor, with a smaller conduit to the power source that does not include an air vent. From January to June 2010, 98% of all LVADs implanted were of continuous flow design.[18]

A third generation of axial flow pumps is under development. These devices provide continuous flow using an impeller suspended either electromagnetically or hydrodynamically. The HeartWare ventricular assist system (HeartWare International Inc, Framingham, MA, USA) is a small, durable, centrifugal flow pump implanted directly in the left ventricular apex and contained within the pericardial space. Aaronson and colleagues[19] recently reported results from a multicenter prospective trial of 140 patients undergoing implantation of the HeartWare as a bridge to transplant. The study's primary composite end point included the proportion of patients alive, transplanted, or explanted for recovery, and without device replacement at 180 days. Results demonstrated noninferiority compared with contemporaneous controls receiving support by currently approved continuous flow LVADs (HeartMate II; Thoratec, Pleasanton, CA, USA). The new device also seems to be associated with a lower infection rate. Although promising, these devices are not yet FDA approved.

OUTCOMES OF MECHANICAL SUPPORT

Infectious complications associated with LVAD placement remain common, although the rate has improved with the newer devices.[20–22] The Interagency Registry for Mechanical Circulatory Support (INTERMACS) started as a collaboration among the National Heart, Lung, and Blood Institute, the Center for Medicaid and Medicare Services (CMS), the FDA, and clinical providers working with VADs. All institutions with CMS approval for mechanical circulatory support as destination therapy must provide clinical data to INTERMACS. Because INTERMACS only collects data on FDA-approved devices, there is little information available on the newest devices.

The second INTERMACS report includes data on devices implanted from June 2006 to March 2009, specifically 1092 primary LVADs and 66 nonprimary LVADs; 564 of these were continuous flow devices. Actuarial survival in the primary LVAD cohort (including both device types) was 83% at 6 months, 74% at 1 year, and 55% at 2 years. Other than heart failure, infection accounted for the leading cause of death and was identified as the cause of 16% of deaths due to LVAD implantation. Of the 69 deaths that occurred within 1 month of implantation, 6 were caused by infection (8.7%). Beyond 1 month, 25 of 122 deaths were infection related (20.5%). Infections accounted for 12.9% of all deaths in bridge-to-transplant patients (N = 54), 17.4% of bridge-to-candidacy patients (N = 92), and 15.4% of destination therapy patients (N = 39).[20]

In terms of overall rates, there were 17.46 infections per 100 patient-months during the first 12 months after implant. The rates varied between generations of device, with 28.9 infections per 100 months in the pulsatile devices (N = 406) and 11.8 infections per 100 months in the continuous flow devices (N = 548) ($P<.0001$).[20] Besides the INTERMACS data, results from a 2009 trial by Slaughter and colleagues[21] offer additional comparisons of infectious complications between older and newer LVAD technology. Investigators randomized patients with advanced heart failure who were ineligible for transplantation to receive either a newer continuous flow device (N = 134) or an older pulsatile flow device (N = 66). Besides improved probability of survival free from stroke and device failure at 2 years, treatment with a continuous flow LVAD was associated with a reduction in infectious complications, both device related and nondevice related.

LVAD INFECTIONS

Infection can involve any portion of an LVAD, including the surgical site, driveline, pocket, and pump. The approach to treatment varies depending on location and severity of infection.

Most infections involve the percutaneous driveline.[3,4,23–25] This part of the device, which includes the power and ventilation sources, is generally covered in velour to promote adherence to patient tissues. Slow or impaired healing is common and can be caused by several factors, especially trauma because patients mobilize after surgery. After an initial trauma, the driveline may continue to slide. This movement further prevents tissue healing and can even result in the creation of a tract parallel to the driveline, which presents a route of entry for infecting organisms.[26] Driveline infections span a large clinical spectrum from localized infection to widespread complicated disease, including bloodstream infection, endocarditis, and sepsis, and can occur early or late.[24,25]

Driveline infections are frequently the primary source of other LVAD-associated infections. There are newer operative techniques for positioning the driveline (or percutaneous lead) that result in a lower incidence of driveline-associated infections. In the future, a totally implantable device will likely significantly reduce the overall risk of infection by eliminating the driveline as a route of organism entry, although no such devices have been approved to date.[24]

The pump pocket is another potential site of infection. This pocket usually consists of a peritoneal space formed below the lateral rectus but can also be formed intra-abdominally. Although a large portion of pump pocket infections are believed to originate from a driveline source, inoculation of this site can occur during or after surgery, including secondary to surgical trauma or hematoma formation.[27] Biofilms on the device material are proposed to play a role in pathogenesis, and it is thought that organisms are protected from host immunity in these areas of relatively poor perfusion, which are generally scarred and walled off.[28,29] Systemic manifestations and disseminated spread from pocket infections are common, although the onset of such infections is often insidious. Some of the newer devices are now positioned within the pericardium, so a pump pocket is no longer necessary (and pocket infection does not occur).[19]

LVAD-related endocarditis can be particularly difficult to manage and occurs when the inner portions of the device are infected.[30] This infection can be caused by ascending pump or driveline infections, bacteremia, fungemia, or can be secondary to other health care–associated infections from urinary or pulmonary sources.

Microbiology

The microbiology of LVAD-associated infections includes the entire range of organisms, although gram-positive pathogens (especially *Staphylococcus aureus* and coagulase-negative staphylococcus) tend to predominate.[6,31] Enterococcal infections are also common, as are gram-negative bacilli, including *Pseudomonas*, *Klebsiella*, and *Enterobacter*.[6] Selection of antimicrobial-resistant flora can result from lengthy hospitalizations and extensive antimicrobial use among this medically complex patient population.[23]

Using INTERMACS data from 2006 to 2008, Holman and colleagues[32] reported that most infections related to mechanical cardiac support devices (87%) were bacterial, with the remainder associated with fungal (9%), viral (1%), protozoal (0.3%), or unknown (2%) causes. Driveline infections are primarily caused by staphylococcal species from skin flora, which may be facilitated by binding of microbial surface components recognizing adhesive matrix molecules to device components.[33] Fungal organisms also play an important role in LVAD infections, most notably *Candida* species, and carry high mortality risk.[2,6,34–36] Risk of fungal infection has been shown to have a significant association with total parenteral nutrition and does not seem to decrease with fungal prophylaxis. Although uncommon, *Aspergillus* infection is described and is universally fatal.[36]

Clinical Manifestations

LVAD infections frequently present in an occult manner with few signs or symptoms. Determining the source or even the presence of infection can be vexing. Common clinical findings such as fever, leukocytosis, as well as wound-related signs, including drainage, necrosis, bleeding, erythema, and pain, are neither sensitive nor specific,[37] and positive cultures may or may not represent clinical disease. Varied presentation, complicated patient population, exposure of patients to broad-spectrum antimicrobials, and prolonged hospital stays combine to impede and delay diagnosis of LVAD-related infection. Given the clinical importance of infection-associated morbidity and mortality and the growing need for meaningful comparison of outcomes among centers, the International Society for Heart and Lung Transplantation (ISHLT) recently published consensus-based guidelines that provide definitions of VAD-specific, VAD-related, and non-VAD infections among patients receiving support.[38]

Infections occur most commonly within the first 3 months of device implantation,[39–41] with risk of severe infection and sepsis peaking at 1 month. Although cumulative risk of device infection increases the longer the device remains in place, the incidence of infection decreases significantly after 3 months.[1]

Driveline infections can be particularly elusive and may simply present with wound dehiscence, poor driveline integration, or persistent serous drainage. The onset of pump pocket infections can also be insidious, with presentation often delayed until systemic spread occurs with resultant bloodstream infection; leukocytosis and fever generally occur late.[42]

LVAD-associated endocarditis carries a high mortality[43] and presents similar to prosthetic valve endocarditis, with clinical manifestations ranging from asymptomatic infection to classic signs and symptoms, including fever, positive blood cultures, and systemic embolic phenomena. Bleeding within the device, hematoma formation, inlet or outflow obstruction, or device malfunction can also be suggestive of endocarditis. Some patients with more subacute infection do not develop significant fever and may instead present with chronic nonspecific symptoms such as weight loss, night sweats, and low-grade increase in temperature.

Risk Factors

A variety of host, device, and operative characteristics predispose to LVAD infection. Device-related risk factors seem to be correlated with increased size and surface area of the device,[44] turbulence of flow, and available entry routes for organisms. As noted previously, the driveline is an important source because it maintains a connection between the device and the external environment. Design of effective fully implantable devices may be one way to mitigate infection risk.[45] Turbulent flow and device size have frequently been implicated as infection risks. The smaller continuous flow pumps have fewer movable components and lower overall infection rates. Environmental and operative risk factors include duration of hospitalization and intensive care unit stay, use of indwelling lines and catheters, parenteral nutrition and possibly operation technique/time, and perioperative antimicrobials used.[46]

In terms of patient factors, the severity of heart failure symptoms, as well as the presence of certain comorbid conditions, including diabetes,[43,47,48] hyperglycemia, alcohol use, obesity,[49,50] and renal disease, has been associated with increased infection risk.[23] Older patient age also seems to be associated with increased infection risk.[43] Extended hospital stay and repeat operations have also been associated with LVAD-related bloodstream infections,[45,50] as well as duration of ventilatory support.[1,45,51] As with other surgical infections, poor nutritional state and the presence of indwelling lines and catheters may increase the risk of LVAD infection.

Relative immunosuppression is believed to play a role in LVAD infections, although the exact association is unclear. Immunologic studies suggest that patients with heart failure receiving VAD support may have diminished T-cell response and activation.[52–54]

Diagnosis

The lack of fully standardized criteria for diagnosis of LVAD-associated infection has been problematic.[38] At times, organisms have grown in routine cultures of explanted devices from patients who showed no signs or symptoms of infection, and it remains unclear whether these organisms represent contamination on removal or undiagnosed infection. Different investigators have proposed different diagnostic paradigms, with positive cultures alone or clinical signs plus positive cultures being the most common. Some studies do not specify their criteria, and others separate infections (with clinical symptoms and positive cultures) into different groups based on whether or not the infection was likely to be device related. The recently published ISHLT definitions offer standardization and guidance both clinically and for future investigative work.[38]

When considering infection in a patient with an LVAD, the recommended diagnostic routine includes comprehensive metabolic panel, basic infection workup (chest radiography, urine studies, and culture and Gram stains of any potentially infected sites), blood cultures, and deep tissue swab or biopsy from driveline, pocket, or other potential source where applicable or feasible. The American Heart Association recommends ultrasonography for pocket site infections, and transesophageal echocardiography for endocarditis. Other experts suggest computed tomography to identify fluid collections around the device, but sensitivity and specificity are limited by artifact, and many patients are unable to tolerate contrast administration because of underlying renal insufficiency. Specificity of imaging is also limited by the nuances of discerning a potentially infected fluid pocket from a benign postoperative fluid collection. Nuclear medicine studies such as tagged white blood cell scans are sometimes done, but their usefulness remains unclear.

LVAD infection not only poses immediate morbidity and mortality but also affects candidacy for transplant because active infection carries significant risk in the setting of the substantial immunosuppression required after cardiac transplantation. Like many device or prosthesis infections, definitive treatment involves device removal, which is often impossible without concurrent transplantation. Although some studies suggest that device-related infections do not reduce survival to transplant, and many have described successful transplant in the setting of device-associated infection and mediastinitis, there remains a high associated mortality and infections can persist after organ transplantation. There is some evidence of an increase in early posttransplant mortality in patients with LVAD infections, but most studies have shown relatively low rates of infection recurrence and no difference in long-term survival after transplant.[43,47,55–58]

Treatment

Although cultures and other workup are pending, the current treatment recommendations for suspected LVAD infection includes empiric broad-spectrum antimicrobials to cover likely pathogens with consideration given to institutional infection patterns, resistance data, and individual patients' prior microbiology and antimicrobial history. Whenever possible, final therapy should be based on culture results. For localized driveline or surgical site infections (SSIs), coverage is often initiated with gram-positive (staphylococcal) coverage alone. Gram-negative coverage is often added for pump pocket infections or deeper wound infections. Regardless of initial agent, relapse is common and infections frequently progress.

Pump pocket infections with fluid collections require drainage, and some infections have been successfully treated with antimicrobial-impregnated beads. Other approaches have included use of an omental or muscle flap to wrap the pocket and help limit infection spread or vacuum-assisted closure therapy.[59,60] Antimicrobials should be used in combination with aggressive wound care and/or debridement where applicable. LVAD explantation with or without subsequent transplantation remains the definitive treatment of significant device-related infection but presents high morbidity and mortality, and the risk of infection relapse remains.[23,55]

Prevention

There is evidence that the overall rates of LVAD infection are decreasing, which may be due to improved patient selection, improved devices, improved transplant team experience, as well as appropriate perioperative antimicrobial prophylaxis. The general principles of SSI prevention also apply to decreasing the risk of LVAD infection, including procedure-related strategies that focus on reducing microbial inoculum and preventing surgical site contamination.[61]

Specific evidence-based interventions include preparation of the surgical site with an appropriate antiseptic agent, proper sterilization and disinfection of equipment, minimizing traffic in the operating room, and use of appropriate ventilation systems. Other approaches address modifiable patient-related factors such as tight perioperative blood glucose control for patients with diabetes.

Systemic antimicrobial prophylaxis is routinely given before LVAD implantation, although the specific agents and duration of use vary widely among institutions. In a recent survey of LVAD surgical infection prophylaxis (SIP) practices, some centers reported routine broad coverage with 4 drug regimens (usually fluconazole with 3 other antimicrobials), whereas others used vancomycin alone. The duration of use also varied, with most centers reporting use for somewhere between 24 and 72 hours postoperatively.[62] This small study highlights the wide variability in SIP regimens across institutions, underscoring the lack of consensus regarding best practices. In addition to systemic antimicrobials, there may be a larger role for chlorhexidine bathing to prevent LVAD infection, particularly regarding the driveline. Several recent studies demonstrate the benefits of chlorhexidine bathing among patients with central venous catheters.[63,64] A modified strategy may help prevent SSIs among LVAD recipients.

There have been several published reports regarding procedural mechanisms to decrease infection risk, including maintaining a low-traffic environment in the operating room, high-efficiency particulate air filters, clean scrub, and covering any exposed hair. Wrapping the pump and driveline in antibiotic-soaked laparotomy pads has also been proposed. Mupirocin ointments to eliminate nasal colonization and chlorhexidine washes are widely used, but data supporting these are limited.

The VADs themselves undergo frequent design changes aimed at mitigating infection; among these have been the use of antimicrobial-impregnated drivelines, using sulfadiazine, chlorhexidine, or triclosan, and use of specialized materials (such as Dacron or Hemashield) to augment integration of device components into host tissues. Tunneling of the driveline contralateral to the pump pocket lengthens the subcutaneous course with the aim of slowing or impeding movement of organisms from the external environment to the pump pocket. The driveline exit site is secured well with an occlusive dressing to prevent organism entry.

Placement of the pump intra-abdominally rather than intraperitoneally has been proposed to decrease infections. However, this placement may increase other complications, such as visceral damage, and may be more technically difficult to perform.[27] To improve safety, some centers are using synthetic pouches to protect the viscera from the working parts of the device.

Postoperative recommendations have included early extubation, aggressive pulmonary toilet, and removal of all indwelling lines and catheters as early as is feasible. Daily cleansing and dressing changes under sterile conditions are recommended, and some have even recommended dressings containing silver to further prevent microbial growth, but this is not standard procedure. Rehabilitation and nutrition play an important role in immunity and wound healing, and stabilization of the driveline along with patient education on wound care and trauma avoidance should be discussed with patients and their families.

SUMMARY

Although LVAD support is associated with improved survival and quality of life, infectious complications remain a major limitation, particularly for destination use. Improvements in device design (smaller size, continuous instead of pulsatile flow, and so forth) have resulted in lower rates of infection. Because the number of patients receiving long-term mechanical support continues to burgeon, additional efforts to determine optimal approaches for treatment and prevention of LVAD-associated infection remain critical.

REFERENCES

1. Gordon RJ, Quagliarello B, Lowy FD. Ventricular assist device-related infections. Lancet Infect Dis 2006;7:426–37.
2. Aslam S, Hernandez M, Thornby J, et al. Risk factors and outcomes of fungal ventricular-assist device infections. Clin Infect Dis 2010;50:664–71.
3. Argenziano M, Catanese KA, Moazami N, et al. The influence of infection on survival and successful transplantation in patients with left ventricular assist devices. J Heart Lung Transplant 1997;16:822–31.
4. Bentz B, Hupcey JE, Polomano RC, et al. A retrospective study of left ventricular assist device-related infections. J Cardiovasc Manag 2004;15:9–16.
5. Cabell CH, Heidenreich PA, Chu VH, et al. Increasing rates of cardiac device infections among Medicare beneficiaries: 1990-1999. Am Heart J 2004;147: 582–6.
6. Gordon SM, Schmitt SK, Jacobs M, et al. Nosocomial bloodstream infections in patients with implantable left ventricular assist devices. Ann Thorac Surg 2001; 72:725–30.
7. Roger VL, Go AS, Lloyd-Jones DM, et al. Heart disease and stroke statistics— 2011 update: a report from the American Heart Association. Circulation 2011; 123(4):e18–209.

8. Writing Group Members, Lloyd-Jones D, Adams RJ, et al. Heart disease and stroke statistics—2010 update: a report from the American Heart Association. Circulation 2010;121:e46–215.

9. Johnson MR, Meyer KH, Haft J, et al. Heart transplantation in the United States, 1999-2008. Am J Transplant 2010;10:1035–46.

10. National Heart, Lung and Blood Institute [Online]. Available at: http://www.nhlbi. nih.gov/health/dci/Diseases/ht/ht_before.html. Accessed July 31, 2011.

11. Merion RM. 2009 SRTR report on the state of transplantation. Am J Transplant 2010;10:959–60.

12. Dembitsky WP, Tector AJ, Park S, et al. Left ventricular assist device performance with long-term circulatory support: lessons from the REMATCH trial. Ann Thorac Surg 2004;78:2123–9.

13. Young JB. Healing the heart with ventricular assist device therapy: mechanisms of cardiac recovery. Ann Thorac Surg 2001;71:S210–9.

14. Bruckner BA, Stetson SJ, Perez-Verdia A, et al. Regression of fibrosis and hypertrophy in failing myocardium following mechanical circulatory support. J Heart Lung Transplant 2001;20:457–64.

15. Heerdt PM, Holmes JW, Cai B, et al. Chronic unloading by left ventricular assist device reverses contractile dysfunction and alters gene expression in end-stage heart failure. Circulation 2000;102:2713–9.

16. Levin HR, Oz MC, Chen JM, et al. Reversal of chronic ventricular dilation in patients with end-stage cardiomyopathy by prolonged mechanical unloading. Circulation 1995;91:2717–20.

17. Westaby S, Jin XY, Katsumata T, et al. Mechanical support in dilated cardiomyopathy: signs of early left ventricular recovery. Ann Thorac Surg 1997;64:1303–8.

18. Kirklin JK, Naftel DC, Kormos RL, et al. Third INTERMACS annual report: the evolution of destination therapy in the United States. J Heart Lung Transplant 2010;30:115–23.

19. Aaronson KD, Slaughter MS, McGee E, et al. Evaluation of the HeartWare HVAD left ventricular assist device system for the treatment of advanced heart failure: results of the ADVANCE bridge to transplant trial. Circulation 2010;122:2216.

20. Kirklin JK, Naftel DC, Kormos RL, et al. Second INTERMACS annual report: more than 1000 primary left ventricular assist device implants. J Heart Lung Transplant 2010;29:1–10.

21. Slaughter MS, Rogers JG, Milano CA, et al. Advanced heart failure treated with continuous-flow left ventricular assist device. N Engl J Med 2009;361: 2241–51.

22. Starling RC, Naka Y, Boyle AJ, et al. Results of the post-U.S. Food and Drug Administration-approval study with a continuous flow left ventricular assist device as a bridge to heart transplantation: a prospective study using the INTERMACS. J Am Coll Cardiol 2011;57:1890–8.

23. Malani PN, Dyke DB, Pagani FD, et al. Nosocomial infections in left ventricular assist device recipients. Clin Infect Dis 2002;34:1295–300.

24. Chinn R, Dembitsky W, Eaton L, et al. Multicenter experience: prevention and management of left ventricular assist device infections. ASAIO J 2005;51: 461–70.

25. Zierer A, Melby SJ, Voeller RK, et al. Late-onset driveline infections: the Achilles' heel of prolonged left ventricular assist device support. Ann Thorac Surg 2007; 84:515–20.

26. Pasque MK, Hanselman T, Shelton K, et al. Surgical management of Novacor drive-line exit site infections. Ann Thorac Surg 2002;74:1267–8.

27. Costantini TW, Taylor JH, Beilman GJ. Abdominal complications of ventricular assist device placement. Surg Infect 2005;6:409–18.
28. Holman WL. Microbiology of infection in mechanical circulatory support. Int J Artif Organs 2007;30:764–70.
29. Padera RF. Infection in ventricular assist devices: the role of biofilm. Cardiovasc Pathol 2006;15:264–70.
30. Holman WL, Skinner JL, Waites KB, et al. Infection during circulatory support with ventricular assist devices. Ann Thorac Surg 1999;68:711–6.
31. Weyand M, Hermann M, Kondruweit M, et al. Clinical impact of infections in left ventricular assist device recipients: the importance of site and organism. Transplant Proc 1997;29:3327–9.
32. Holman WL, Pae WE, Teutenberg JJ, et al. INTERMACS: interval analysis of registry data. J Am Coll Cardiol 2009;208:755–61.
33. Arrecubieta C, Asai T, Bayern M, et al. The role of *Staphylococcus aureus* adhesins in the pathogenesis of ventricular assist device-related infections. J Infect Dis 2006;193:1109–19.
34. Nurozler F, Argenziano M, Oz MC, et al. Fungal left ventricular assist device endocarditis. Ann Thorac Surg 2001;71:614–8.
35. Shoham S, Shaffer R, Sweet L, et al. Candidemia in patients with ventricular assist devices. Clin Infect Dis 2007;44:e9–12.
36. Bagdasarian NG, Malani AN, Pagani FD, et al. Fungemia associated with left ventricular assist device support. J Card Surg 2009;24:763–5.
37. Sivaratnam K, Duggan JM. Left ventricular assist device infections: three case reports and a review of the literature. ASAIO J 2002;48:2–7.
38. Hannan MM, Husain S, Mattner F, et al. Working formulation for the standardization of definitions of infections in patients using ventricular assist devices. J Heart Lung Transplant 2011;30:375–84.
39. Holman WL, Kirklin JK, Naftel DC, et al. Infection after implantation of pulsatile mechanical circulatory support devices. J Thorac Cardiovasc Surg 2010;139:632–1636.
40. Holman WL, Park SJ, Long JW, et al. Infection in permanent circulatory support: experience from the REMATCH trial. J Heart Lung Transplant 2004;23:1359–65.
41. Karchmer AW, Longworth DL. Infections of intracardiac devices. Infect Dis Clin North Am 2002;16:477–505.
42. Holman WL, Rayburn BK, McGiffin DC, et al. Infection in ventricular assist devices: prevention and treatment. Ann Thorac Surg 2003;75:S48–57.
43. Monkowski DH, Axelrod P, Fekete T, et al. Infections associated with ventricular assist devices: epidemiology and effect on prognosis after transplantation. Transpl Infect Dis 2007;9:114–20.
44. Pae WE, Connell JM, Adelowo A, et al. Does total implantability reduce infection with the use of a left ventricular assist device? The LionHeart experience in Europe. J Heart Lung Transplant 2007;26:219–29.
45. Myers TJ, Khan T, Frazier OH. Infectious complications associated with ventricular assist systems. ASAIO J 2000;46:S28–36.
46. Lietz K, Long JW, Kfoury AG, et al. Outcomes of left ventricular assist device implantation as destination therapy in the post-REMATCH era: implications for patient selection. Circulation 2007;116:497–505.
47. Simon D, Fischer S, Grossman A, et al. Left ventricular assist device-related infection: treatment and outcome. Clin Infect Dis 2005;40:1108–15.
48. Bhama JK, Rayappa S, Zaldonis D, et al. Impact of abdominal complications on outcome after mechanical circulatory support. Ann Thorac Surg 2010;89: 522–8.

49. Raymond AL, Kfoury AG, Bishop CJ, et al. Obesity and left ventricular assist device driveline exit site infection. ASAIO J 2010;56:57–60.
50. Poston RS, Husain S, Sorce D, et al. LVAD bloodstream infections: therapeutic rationale for transplantation after LVAD infection. J Heart Lung Transplant 2003; 22:914–21.
51. Herrmann M, Weyand M, Greshake B, et al. Left ventricular assist device infection is associated with increased mortality but is not a contraindication to transplantation. Circulation 1997;95:814–7.
52. Ankersmit HJ, Tugulea S, Spanier T, et al. Activation-induced T-cell death and immune dysfunction after implantation of left-ventricular assist device. Lancet 1999;354:550–5.
53. Itescu S, John R. Interactions between the recipient immune system and the left ventricular assist device surface: immunological and clinical implications. Ann Thorac Surg 2003;75:S58–65.
54. Kimball PM, Flattery M, McDougan F, et al. Cellular immunity impaired among patients on left ventricular assist device for 6 months. Ann Thorac Surg 2008; 85:1656–61.
55. Fischer SA, Trenholme GM, Costanzo MR, et al. Infectious complications in left ventricular assist device recipients. Clin Infect Dis 1997;24:18–23.
56. Morgan JA, Park Y, Oz MC, et al. Device related infections while on left ventricular assist device support do not adversely impact bridging to transplant or post-transplant survival. ASAIO J 2003;49:748–50.
57. Myers TJ, McGee MG, Zeluff BJ, et al. Frequency and significance of infections in patients receiving prolonged LVAD support. ASAIO Trans 1991;37:283–5.
58. Schulman AR, Martens TP, Russo MJ, et al. Effect of left ventricular assist device infection on post-transplant outcomes. J Heart Lung Transplant 2009;28:237–42.
59. Baradarian S, Stahovich M, Krause S, et al. Case series: clinical management of persistent mechanical assist device driveline drainage using vacuum-assisted closure therapy. ASAIO J 2006;52:354–6.
60. Garatti A, Giuseppe B, Russo CF, et al. Drive-line exit-site infection in a patient with axial-flow pump support: successful management using vacuum-assisted therapy. J Heart Lung Transplant 2007;26:956–9.
61. Anderson DJ, Kaye KS, Classen D, et al. Strategies to prevent surgical site infections in acute care hospitals. Infect Control Hosp Epidemiol 2008;29:S51–61.
62. Walker PC, Depestel DD, Miles NA, et al. Surgical infection prophylaxis practices for left ventricular assist device implantation. J Card Surg 2011;26:440–3.
63. Popovich KJ, Hota B, Hayes R, et al. Effectiveness of routine patient cleansing with chlorhexidine gluconate for infection prevention in the medical intensive care unit. Infect Control Hosp Epidemiol 2009;30:959–63.
64. Munoz-Price LS, Hota B, Stemer A, et al. Prevention of bloodstream infection by use of daily chlorhexidine baths for patients at a long-term acute care hospital. Infect Control Hosp Epidemiol 2009;30:1031–5.

Central Nervous System Device Infections

Edward Stenehjem, MD, Wendy S. Armstrong, MD*

KEYWORDS

• Ventriculostomy • Deep brain stimulator • Infection
• Meningitis • Ventriculitis

CEREBROSPINAL FLUID DIVERSION WITH VENTRICULOSTOMIES: VENTRICULOSTOMY-RELATED INFECTIONS

The first operative procedure for hydrocephalus was recorded in the medical literature by Dandy[1] in 1922. Since then, cerebrospinal fluid (CSF) diversion techniques have become common neurosurgical procedures. Ventriculostomy catheters (also known as external ventricular drains or EVDs) serve an increasingly important role in the neurosurgical intensive care unit (ICU). These temporary devices, which permit therapeutic CSF drainage while monitoring intracranial pressure, are used broadly; after closed head injuries, intracranial hemorrhage including subarachnoid hemorrhage (SAH), intracerebral hemorrhage (ICH), and intraventricular hemorrhage (IVH), or for hydrocephalus due to obstructing mass lesions. As with any device, however, EVDs carry a risk of infection, in this case ventriculomeningitis, in an often critically ill and complex patient population.

Ventriculomeningitis may result from contamination of the drain during insertion, contamination of the drain system during routine care and manipulation, colonization of the drain at the insertion site by skin flora, or infection of the drain and CSF as a result of a surgical-site infection. Prevention efforts can be targeted to these potential routes of infection.

Incidence

The incidence of ventriculomeningitis due to EVD catheters is estimated to range from 0% to greater than 20%, but varies widely depending on the definition of infection used and the clinical characteristics of the study population. A large meta-analysis evaluated 23 major studies of ventriculostomy use and encompassed 5733 EVD

The authors have nothing to disclose.
Division of Infectious Diseases, Emory University School of Medicine, 49 Jesse Hill Junior Drive, Atlanta, GA 30303, USA
* Corresponding author.
E-mail address: wsarmst@emory.edu

Infect Dis Clin N Am 26 (2012) 89–110
doi:10.1016/j.idc.2011.09.006
0891-5520/12/$ – see front matter © 2012 Elsevier Inc. All rights reserved.

insertions among 5261 patients. This study found the cumulative rate of positive CSF cultures was 8.80% per patient or 8.08% per EVD placement.[2] As was noted in other reports, studies that defined infection with clinical indicators in addition to a positive CSF culture showed a lower risk of infection of 6.62% per patient or 6.10% per EVD.

Risk Factors

Understanding the risk factors for infection can help guide prevention efforts (**Box 1**). Factors studied include the indication for catheter placement, duration of catheterization, difference in placement technique, antimicrobial use, and frequency of manipulation and sampling. Early in the use of ventriculostomy catheters, IVH and SAH were associated with a higher risk of infection than were other indications. In 1988, Sundbarg and colleagues[3] reported on 648 patients who were subject to prolonged ventricular fluid pressure recording, and found an infection rate of 10% among those with SAH and 13.2% among "other spontaneous hemorrhage." By contrast, the investigators reported a rate of 0% to 2.6% for all other diagnosis, which included tumors, trauma, nonhemorrhage-related hydrocephalus, and miscellaneous indications. Multiple other reports have shown a similar association with hemorrhagic parameters in the CSF and an elevated risk of infection.[4,5] By contrast, in 2008 Hoefnagel and colleagues[6] reported on a retrospective study of 228 patients requiring EVD placement and found no association with infection and IVH. This trend has been duplicated in other retrospective reviews.[7,8] An expanded focus on infection control and sterile manipulation may be contributing to this discrepancy. A heightened suspicion for CSF infection is still warranted among patients with SAH or IVH.

Duration

A lengthy debate regarding the duration of EVD placement and risk of infection has been ongoing since Mayhall and colleagues[5] published their work in 1984. In this prospective study the investigators found a significant increase in ventriculostomy-related infections (VRI) after 5 days of catheterization. Based on these data, the investigators recommended prophylactic removal and reinsertion at day 5 if continued monitoring was needed. Multiple studies have subsequently evaluated duration as a risk factor for infection, with conflicting results,[6-15] and prophylactic removal and reinsertion has proved not to be beneficial.[4,11,16]

Box 1
Risk factors for ventriculostomy-related infections

- Intraventricular hemorrhage
- Subarachnoid hemorrhage
- Depressed cranial fracture
- CSF leak from fracture or ventriculostomy site
- Neurosurgical operation
- Duration of catheterization
- Severity of underlying illness
- Systemic infection
- Frequent manipulation and sampling of drainage system
- Catheter irrigation

A follow-up to the original Mayhall study used daily infection rates to further analyze the relationship between VRI and duration of catheterization. This large retrospective study evaluated 584 patients who had undergone ventriculostomy placement. Sixty-one patients subsequently developed infection (10.4%). The investigators noted that the daily infection rate rose during the monitoring period and reached a peak at day 10. After day 10 there was only one infection in the 42 patients still at risk.[4] These data have been replicated in two additional studies in two different populations of patients.[17,18] Data on late infection are very difficult to interpret, due to the small numbers of patients with prolonged EVD catheterization. Taken together, although the results are conflicting, the data support an increased risk of early infection in the first 10 days after ventriculostomy placement followed by a markedly decreased risk of infection. This finding suggests that a significant proportion of infections may originate from the insertion procedure. The lack of a progressive increase in the rate of infection with duration of catheter days after day 10 in most studies indicates that delayed contamination associated with EVD care may play less of a role than originally thought. Even though the data are mixed on the influence duration has on infection risk, timely removal of invasive devices remains the safest approach to prevention of infection.

CSF leakage from the ventriculostomy placement site,[12] reinsertions of EVDs due to malfunction,[8] catheter irrigation,[5] frequent CSF sampling,[6] and severity of underlying illness (including systemic infections)[4,19] are all associated with higher rates of ventriculomeningitis. A higher index of suspicion should be maintained when a patient has multiple risk factors for infection.

Microbiology

The most commonly found pathogens in VRIs traditionally have been skin flora.[3] However, gram-negative pathogens are increasingly recognized as the etiologic agent.[11,12,20] For example, both Camacho and colleagues[20] (Brazil) and Lo and colleagues[11] (Australia) reported *Acinetobacter* as the most common etiologic agent in their recent studies, whereas Schade and colleagues[9] (Netherlands) and Flibotte and colleagues[21] (United States) reported staphylococci as being the most common pathogen in VRI. This variability in microbiology is likely due to regional antimicrobial prescribing patterns affecting the local flora and to geographic differences (**Table 1**), and directly affects the selection of empiric anti-infective therapy. VRIs caused by fungi have been reported in the literature, but generally account for a small fraction of all cases.[14,21]

Diagnosis

The difficulty in comparing studies of VRIs stems in large part from variability in how infection is defined. The most widely used definition of hospital-acquired meningitis/ventriculitis is the one proposed by the Centers for Disease Control and Prevention (CDC) and the National Healthcare Safety Network (NHSN).[22] The definition states patients must meet at least one of the following two criteria:

1. Patient has organisms cultured from CSF
2. Patient has at least one of the following signs or symptoms with no other recognized cause: fever (>38°C), headache, stiff neck, meningeal signs, cranial nerve signs, or irritability *and* at least 1 of the following: (a) increased white cells, elevated protein, and/or decreased glucose in CSF; (b) organisms seen on Gram stain of CSF; (c) organisms cultured from blood; (d) positive antigen test of CSF, blood, or urine; (e) diagnostic single antibody titer (IgM) or fourfold increase in paired

Table 1
Microbiology of ventriculostomy-related infections

Study, Ref. Year	Country	No. of Positive Cultures	Coagulase-Negative Staphylococci	S aureus	Acinetobacter	Pseudomonas	Enterobacteriaciae	Other
Camacho et al,[20] 2011	Brazil	22	2 (9%)	1 (5%)	6 (27%)[a]	3 (14%)	7 (32%)	3 (14%)
Chi et al,[8] 2010	Taiwan	35	1 (3%)	2 (6%)	6 (17%)	9 (26%)	7 (20%)	10 (29%)
Scheithauer et al,[14] 2010	Germany	21[b]	9 (43%)	4 (19%)	1 (5%)		6 (29%)	1 (5%)
Lo et al,[11] 2007	Australia	25	4 (16%)	2 (8%)	10 (40%)	1 (4%)	4 (16%)	4 (16%)
Orsi et al,[86] 2006	Italy	11	2 (18%)	1 (9%)		4 (36%)	1 (9%)	3 (27%)
Korinek et al,[10] 2005	France	57	44 (77%)	4 (7%)	1 (2%)	1 (2%)	1 (2%)	6 (11%)
Arabi et al,[18] 2005	Saudi Arabia	22[c]	3 (14%)	1 (5%)	6 (27%)	2 (9%)	4 (18%)	3 (14%)
Bota et al,[87] 2005	Belgium	58	21 (36%)	18 (31%)	2 (3%)	3 (5%)	12 (21%)	2 (3%)
Schade et al,[9] 2005	Netherlands	14	8 (57%)	3 (21%)			1 (7%)	2 (14%)
Flibotte et al,[21] 2004	USA	17[b]	12 (71%)	1 (6%)		1 (6%)	1 (6%)	1 (6%)
Lyke et al,[12] 2001	USA	11	2 (18%)				9 (82%)	
Sundbarg et al,[3] 1988	Sweden	27	16 (59%)	4 (15%)	2 (7%)		1 (4%)	4 (15%)
Mayhall et al,[5] 1984	USA	19	6 (32%)	1 (5%)	2 (10%)		8 (42%)	2 (11%)

[a] One-half were resistant to carbapenem antibiotics.
[b] Included 1 case of fungal infection.
[c] Included 3 cases of fungal infection.

sera (IgG) for pathogen *and* if diagnosis is made antemortem, physician institutes appropriate antimicrobial therapy.

Although very sensitive, this definition can lead to confusion in practice. The first criterion does not distinguish between infection, colonization, or contamination, and may lead clinicians to overtreat patients for presumed ventriculitis. Studies that use this definition may include patients with a spectrum of disease from contamination to colonization to true ventriculitis, complicating the generalizability of the results. The clinical features defined in criterion (2) are equally controversial. Patients with ICH/ischemia or recent neurosurgery frequently show signs of aseptic meningitis with fever, headache, stiff neck, and/or meningeal signs. In critically ill patients who are often intubated and sedated, these clinical signs and symptoms may be unreliable or impossible to assess. In addition, CSF parameters can be very abnormal in patients with ICH.

In an attempt to achieve further clarity, Lozier and colleagues[2] proposed a diagnostic method that differentiates contamination, colonization, and infection, and focuses on identifying clinically relevant infections. Contamination is defined as an isolated positive CSF culture (and/or Gram stain) with CSF glucose, protein, and cell count in the expected range. Colonization is defined as repeated positive CSF cultures (and/or Gram stain) with normal CSF profile without clinical symptoms other than possible fever. Progressive decline in CSF glucose, increasing CSF protein, and advancing CSF pleocytosis with one or more positive CSF cultures (and/or Gram stain) define VRI. Similar patterns of CSF parameters that lack positive microbiologic data signify a suspected VRI.

Although the Lozier definition uses CSF and clinical parameters in diagnosing infection, a strict definition of what constitutes abnormal CSF parameters cannot be identified, due to the variability in CSF profiles among patients with CNS disease.[23,24] Muttaiyah and colleagues[25] compared CSF glucose and protein, daily maximum temperature, and Glasgow Coma Scale (GCS) in patients with VRIs and those with EVDs in place and no infection. The investigators found no difference between the groups in CSF protein, temperature, or GCS in this retrospective, laboratory-based study. The VRI group did have statistically significant lower CSF glucose on average. Of note, of the isolates identified as contaminants as per the Lozier definition, none had a positive CSF Gram stain (compared with 45% in those with VRI), all were isolated in a single culture (66% of VRIs grew in multiple cultures), coagulase-negative *Staphylococcus* was the most common organism, and none of the contaminants were gram-negative rods.[25] Schade and colleagues[26] performed a well-designed matched case-control study analyzing the predictive and diagnostic value of routine CSF analysis among a cohort of 230 consecutive patients with EVDs. The results showed that CSF cell count, glucose, and protein concentrations in patients with VRIs were comparable with those in patients with no infection. While controlling for duration of drainage and using univariate regression analysis and receiver-operating characteristic curves, the investigators were unable to identify a significant predictive or diagnostic value for any commonly used CSF parameter. Evaluating the results of the same patient longitudinally also failed to predict or recognize an infection. These findings led the investigators to propose that routine use of CSF parameters has no additional value for diagnosing VRI and that the diagnosis of VRI can be based only on the results of microbiologic cultures.

Multiple other laboratory parameters have been evaluated as potential diagnostic aids in VRI. Pfausler and colleagues[27] hypothesized that the ratio of CSF leukocytes to erythrocytes should parallel the leukocyte to erythrocyte ratio in the serum among those without infection. In a study of 13 patients with IVH, following the cell index ([leukocytes(CSF)/erythrocytes(CSF)]/[leukocytes(serum)/erythrocytes(serum)]) for an increase in the ratio accurately predicted VRI 3 days ahead of conventional methods. The cell index as a single time point showed no predictive value. Although cited frequently as a potential diagnostic tool, these findings have not been validated and were found not to be associated with earlier detection of infection in a subsequent study.[26]

Other parameters such as serum procalcitonin,[28,29] CSF lactate,[30] CSF interleukin-6,[26] and CSF real-time polymerase chain reaction[31] are not yet ready to be implemented in diagnostic algorithms. Lacking a reliable definition of infection, in the majority of cases the diagnosis of VRI effectively will be made based on microbiologic results and be supported by CSF parameters, basic laboratory evaluation, and clinical evaluation.

Management of Ventriculostomy-Related Infections

Antimicrobial therapy

Very few adequately controlled clinical trials have evaluated appropriate treatment strategies for VRIs. Although selecting the most appropriate antimicrobials and initiating them in a timely fashion is the key to successful treatment of VRIs, most recommendations are based on expert opinion, previous experience, and small observational clinical trials. Early and appropriate antimicrobial therapy has been associated with better clinical outcomes in the ICU.[32–34] The agents chosen must be active against the most likely organisms encountered based on local epidemiologic trends, and must achieve adequate concentration in the CNS.

Due to the high rates of nosocomial staphylococci (both coagulase-negative and *Staphylococcus aureus*), vancomycin is routinely given as part of the first-line empiric regimen. However, even with meningeal inflammation, CSF penetration is not guaranteed. In a pharmacokinetics trial vancomycin, 500 mg intravenously every 6 hours, was administered to patients with staphylococcal VRIs. In the 5 patients treated with intravenous vancomycin, the mean serum trough level was 13.29 μg/mL and the CSF concentration never rose above 5 μg/mL. Regardless, all 5 patients were cured and no relapses were observed.[35] Alternative agents to vancomycin must be used in patients with intolerance or allergy, significant comorbidities, and those with resistant pathogens (ie, vancomycin-resistant *Enterococcus*, *S aureus* with elevated minimum inhibitory concentration [MIC]). The oxazolidinone agent linezolid is predominantly bacteriostatic with a broad gram-positive spectrum. In an observational trial of 5 patients with staphylococcal ventriculitis treated with linezolid, 600 mg intravenously every 12 hours, the CSF concentration of linezolid was above the mean inhibitory concentration 99.8% and 57.2% of the time for isolates with MICs of 2 mg/L and 4 mg/L, respectively.[36] These results have been duplicated in other pharmacokinetic studies,[37,38] but minimal clinical outcome data are known with the use of linezolid.[39–42] Due to its inability to cross the blood-brain barrier, daptomycin has not been studied in CNS infections. With methicillin-susceptible isolates, nafcillin would generally be preferred over vancomycin.

Gram-negative infections are also common in VRI and at times account for the majority of isolated pathogens.[20] Along with vancomycin, an antipseudomonal cephalosporin or carbapenem should be used in the initial management of suspected VRI. The decision to use a carbapenem should be based on institutional rates of extended spectrum β-lactamase–producing organisms and local gram-negative susceptibility patterns. Patients with significant penicillin allergies have few options for systemic antimicrobial therapy, as aminoglycosides do not cross the blood-brain barrier effectively. Aztreonam and colistin remain options that have not been well studied.

The optimal treatment for fungal VRI remains unknown. Fluconazole and voriconazole are known to achieve the best levels in the CSF while amphotericin B, itraconazole, and the echinocandins achieve low levels. Nevertheless, most of these agents achieve adequate brain tissue levels and in the case of amphotericin B, there is significant clinical experience suggesting efficacy. As most VRIs are confined to the CSF, perhaps the optimal choice is fluconazole or voriconazole depending on the infecting species.[43]

Intraventricular therapy

Treatment of VRI using intrathecal antimicrobials is challenging, with no reliable clinical data to support their use in adults. There are currently no antimicrobials for intrathecal use approved by the Food and Drug Administration and there is no consensus among the medical community on indications for using the intrathecal route. In addition, there are few data to guide decisions regarding the timing of intrathecal therapy, choice and duration of agents, the role for therapeutic drug monitoring, and whether concomitant systemic therapy should also be administered.

Even with significant publication bias, there are promising results supporting the use of intrathecal therapy in cases of VRI that are difficult to treat. Intrathecal vancomycin has been used to treat methicillin-resistant *S aureus* (MRSA),[35] intrathecal gentamicin has been used to treat gram-negative pathogens,[44] intrathecal daptomycin has been used to treat *Enterococcus faecalis*,[45] and a growing literature supports the use of intrathecal colistin for the treatment of multidrug-resistant (MDR) *Acinetobacter*.[46,47] Despite the lack of data, intrathecal antimicrobial therapy may be considered in the setting of severe ventriculitis, persistently positive CSF cultures despite appropriate intravenous dosing, MDR pathogen requiring a specific antimicrobial that does not achieve target MIC concentrations in the CSF, adverse reaction or systemic comorbidities leading to intolerance of systemic administration of intravenous antimicrobial, and, in rare circumstances, when device removal is not feasible.

The most commonly used intrathecal antimicrobials include vancomycin, aminoglycosides (gentamicin, tobramycin, amikacin), and colistin/polymixin B.[48] Intrathecal amphotericin B has been used extensively in a variety of settings but is associated with significant toxicity, including arachnoiditis and symptoms of chemical meningitis such as headache and vomiting, amongst many others.[49]

The pharmacokinetics of intrathecal antimicrobials have recently been reviewed.[50] Targeting a CSF concentration 10 times the MIC of the pathogen is thought to be adequate to achieve rapid bactericidal killing (inhibitory quotient).[48] Calculating an inhibitory quotient prior to the second dose of intrathecal therapy can ensure adequate dosing, and subsequent doses can be held if the drug concentration remains elevated. In sum, intrathecal antimicrobial therapy may have a role in the treatment of ventriculomeningitis; however, additional safety and efficacy data are required.

Miscellaneous management issues

Duration of antimicrobial therapy, importance of device removal, and timing of internal shunt placement after EVD infection are clinically relevant issues that lack evidence-based answers. Based on existing literature for vascular catheter-related bloodstream infections,[51,52] ventriculostomy catheter removal or exchange is encouraged with all infections when clinically feasible. Device retention can be considered in hemodynamically stable patients with minimal alteration in CSF cell counts and cultures positive for coagulase-negative staphylococci, if the duration of catheterization is anticipated to be short (<3 days) and an internal shunt will not be placed. Removal of the infected catheter is also an important measure when appropriate therapy fails to sterilize the CSF.

Because of the complexity of the patients in the neurologic critical care unit, firm guidelines for duration of therapy for VRIs are difficult to establish. For S aureus, fungi, and gram-negative pathogens, treatment for 10 to 14 days after device removal with negative cultures is usually recommended. Treatment for 7 to 10 days after device removal may often be adequate for coagulase-negative staphylococci. In the authors' opinion, shunt internalization may be performed at the end of therapy without an antimicrobial-free interval if negative cultures have been documented. Longer durations of therapy may be needed based on the clinical situation.

Prevention of Infection

Bundles

The new emphasis on health care–associated infections has led to the study of novel methods to decrease central line–related bloodstream infections, ventilator-associated pneumonia, and catheter-associated urinary tract infections, with encouraging results.[53,54] One of these methods, known as care bundles, groups best practices for a disease process that individually improve care but when applied together result in substantially greater improvement. For example, central line bundles have led to significant improvements in the rate of central line–associated bloodstream infections.[54,55] This same concept has been applied to the placement and maintenance of EVDs.

To tackle unacceptably high levels of EVD-related ventriculitis, Korinek and colleagues[10] in France implemented a standardized EVD placement and care protocol. The protocol called for: (a) strict EVD insertion techniques: all procedures were performed in the operating room, all hair was removed with clippers, and the catheter was tunneled under the skin; (b) strict enforcement of the closed drainage system in the ICU: the drainage bag was emptied only when full, manipulations were strongly discouraged, and rinsing of the catheter was forbidden; and (c) routine cultures were not performed and prophylactic antibiotics were given for emergency cases only. During the study period, 216 EVDs were placed in 175 patients. After protocol implementation, the cumulative infection incidence decreased from 12.2% per patient to 5.7% per patient, and the incidence of infection per procedure declined from 9.9% to 4.6% (both results statistically significant, P values not given).[10] Furthermore, violations of the EVD protocol, when studied prospectively, were associated with increased rates of EVD-related infections.

Another European group motivated by high infection rates developed a bundled protocol for EVD insertion and care. Their protocol was based on 5 pillars: increased awareness of the problem, development and implementation of standard operating procedures in the operating room and during subsequent ICU care, development of a diagnostic and therapeutic algorithm for patients with clinical suspicion of drain-related meningitis, antimicrobial prophylaxis before insertion, and adaptation of the drainage system. Comparing prospective study data from 2004 to 2006 with retrospective control data collected from 2003, a significant reduction in rates of infection was seen, declining from 37% in 2003 to 9% in 2005 and 2006.[56]

These two studies, in addition to others,[57] demonstrate the effectiveness of protocols to ensure standardized care of patients with EVDs. Most hospitals have yet to adopt measures to standardize EVD protocols, but strong consideration should be given to implementation of a bundled approach, especially in high-volume centers.

Antimicrobial prophylaxis

The management of prophylactic antimicrobials in neurosurgical patients with CNS devices is complex, with no standard protocols or well-studied recommendations. Most institutional practices are based on personal experience, and vary considerably between institutions and among providers within an institution. The options for prophylaxis include:

- Periprocedural or prolonged systemic antimicrobials
- Antimicrobial impregnated or non-antimicrobial coated catheters
- Combination treatment with treated catheters and systemic antimicrobials
- No prophylaxis with attention to strict infection control measures

Studies evaluating these options are limited, with varying quality and sample size. In addition, the diverse patient populations, different definitions of infection, variable infection control practices, and different surgical techniques used make comparisons problematic. Meta-analyses should be interpreted with caution.[58]

Systemic antimicrobial prophylaxis

Periprocedural and prolonged antimicrobials were found to have no clinical benefit in most of the initial trials in the 1970s and 1980s. The relevance of these studies is questionable, however, given the changes in the practice of neurosurgery, infection control, and microbiologic trends in the current era. More recently, two prospective cohort studies have been published that evaluated the benefit of periprocedural prophylaxis. In both studies the use of periprocedural cephalosporins showed no benefit in preventing VRI by multivariate analysis.[18,20] Both studies were performed outside of the United States and are limited by a cohort design.

Two studies have also compared the use of periprocedural with prolonged therapy for the entire duration the EVD remains in place. Alleyne and colleagues[59] found no statistical difference between infection rates of the two groups in a single-center, retrospective review. The investigators found a 4.0% infection rate when cefuroxime was given as periprocedural prophylaxis and an infection rate of 3.8% when cefuroxime was given for the duration the EVD was in place. There were no infections with MRSA in either group. Poon and colleagues[60] evaluated the use of periprocedural ampicillin/sulbactam and prolonged therapy (for the duration of EVD placement) with ampicillin/sulbactam and aztreonam. In this trial, the patients with prolonged use of antimicrobials had fewer infectious complications (3% vs 11%); however, the prolonged group had an increase in MRSA and *Candida* infections, and a higher mortality rate once infected.

Antimicrobial impregnated catheters

After antimicrobial impregnated central venous catheters were found to reduce central line colonization and infection rates, these catheters were evaluated for reduction of rates of VRI as well.[61] In 2003, Zabramski and colleagues[62] performed a prospective, randomized controlled trial comparing a minocycline/rifampin-coated EVD with a standard EVD. This well-performed study in adult patients found a reduction of infection from 9.4% to 1.3% with the use of coated catheters. The investigators also found a significant reduction in colonization (36.7% vs 17.9%) with coated catheters.

The Zabramski study was followed by 3 observational trials comparing a clindamycin/rifampin catheter with historical controls. All 3 trials found a significant reduction in infection rates with the antimicrobial impregnated catheter.[63–65] One study also noted the time until infection developed was greater in the antimicrobial-coated catheter group than in the standard group.[63]

At present only two types of antimicrobial impregnated catheters are available, minocycline/rifampin or clindamycin/rifampin, both of which specifically target staphylococcal infections. No difference in efficacy has been found, and institutional preference usually dictates use. Abla and colleagues[66] performed a single-center study comparing the two types of catheter. Each catheter was used in alternating 3-month blocks and patients were followed prospectively. Of the 129 patients enrolled (64 minocycline versus 65 clindamycin), no infections were recorded in either group. Of interest, only 50% of the patients received periprocedural antimicrobial, calling into question the additional contribution of systemic prophylaxis when impregnated catheters are used.

The most convincing study of antimicrobial-impregnated catheters is a longitudinal study comparing infection rates after implementation of a standardized protocol for EVD insertion with and without the use of coated catheters.[67] At a single center in Philadelphia, the baseline rate of VRIs in 2003 was 6.7%. After implementation of a standardized protocol, the infection rate did not change significantly; however, after changing to a clindamycin/rifampin ventricular catheter along with standardized protocols, the rate dropped to 1%. After reverting back to standard catheters, the infection rate rose to 7.6%. Subsequently, minocycline/rifampin catheters in combination with standard protocols were introduced and the infection rate again dropped to 0.9%.

Two concerns have been raised regarding impregnated catheters. First, CSF cultures drawn through a coated catheter could be falsely negative. A group in North Carolina was able to demonstrate decreased colony counts when a standard inoculum of *Staphylococcus epidermidis* was drawn through an antimicrobial impregnated catheter in comparison with a nonimpregnated catheter.[68] Until this issue is resolved, caution should be taken when interpreting CSF culture data from impregnated catheters in order to avoid an inappropriately short duration of antimicrobial therapy.

Second, concerns about development of resistance to drugs used in the impregnated catheters have stimulated in vitro research addressing this issue. In the laboratory, sequential exposure of MRSA, methicillin-sensitive *S aureus,* vancomycin-resistant *Enterococcus*, and methicillin-sensitive *S epidermidis* to a minocycline/rifampin catheter did not induce resistance in any of the isolates, and minimal changes in the MIC were noted after 7 sequential exposures.[69]

Although these data are reassuring, non-antimicrobial substances have been evaluated in hopes of avoiding the resistance issue. Catheters impregnated with silver nanoparticles and insoluble silver salts have previously been studied in vascular and urinary catheters, with mixed results.[70,71] A more recent study compared EVD-associated infection rates with silver-coated catheters with those of standard ventricular catheters.[72] This study demonstrated a reduction in the primary outcome defined as a positive CSF culture, colonization of the catheter tip, or CSF pleocytosis in the silver group compared with standard catheters (18.9% vs 33.7%). As more clinical data become available, silver-coated catheters may become an antimicrobial-sparing option for infection prevention.

There are no standard guidelines for the use of antimicrobial prophylaxis for ventriculostomy placement, and most practice patterns are based on clinical experience and institutional policy. The use of broad-spectrum antibiotics in a prolonged prophylactic fashion can lead to the emergence of resistant organisms and adverse events such as *Clostridium difficile*. From the data available, prolonged use of prophylactic antimicrobials should be avoided while periprocedural prophylaxis may be considered. Antimicrobial-impregnated catheters (with or without periprocedural systemic prophylaxis) appear to be a most promising and effective option, and should be considered in all neurosurgical units.

CSF DIVERSION WITH SHUNTS: SHUNT INFECTIONS

The general principles of VRI can be applied to the diagnosis, management, and prevention of CSF shunt infections. Primary CSF shunts (shunt placement with no prior history of neurosurgical procedures) are most commonly placed in adults to treat idiopathic normal-pressure hydrocephalus. Tumors, SAH, head injury, and IVH are the most common causes requiring secondary shunt surgery (placement after EVD placement or craniotomy). The typical CSF shunt has a proximal segment that enters the lateral ventricle via a burr hole and a distal portion that terminates most commonly in either the peritoneal (ventriculoperitoneal [VP]), pleural, or vascular (ventriculoatrial [VA]) space. The entire shunt is internalized and can be accessed via a subcutaneous ventricular reservoir. Infection rates are similar to those of EVDs, but higher rates are found in patients requiring secondary shunt surgery.[73]

Unique patterns of infection have been observed depending on the location of the distal shunt catheter. Bowel perforation may lead to catheter contamination and retrograde infection with gram-negative pathogens among patients with VP shunts. Patients with VA shunts are at higher risk for infections because of hematogenous seeding of the distal catheter. Shunts may also be infected through the skin from accessing the ventricular reservoir. Colonization at the time of implantation, however, is thought to be the most common source, as the majority of infections occur within 30 days of initial surgery and are due to common skin pathogens including staphylococci.[73,74]

The diagnostic principles of shunt infections are similar to those of VRI. CSF culture, Gram stain, chemistries, and cell count continue to be the diagnostic mainstays. CSF cell counts need to be interpreted with caution, as recent surgery or cerebrovascular accident may lead to an inflammatory reaction. Blood cultures should always be performed in patients with VA shunts and are often positive. It is important for the clinician to be aware that signs and symptoms of shunt infection can manifest only at the distal catheter site and not be typical of ventriculomeningitis. Distal infection may result in pleuritis or peritonitis. Peritoneal signs may range from mild, localized tenderness to symptoms of an acute abdomen. Peritoneal inflammation from a shunt infection may result in encystment of the shunt catheter in an attempt to limit the spread of infection. In these cases CSF findings may be bland. VP shunts with distal occlusion and negative CSF findings must be evaluated for infection at the time of revision. Computed tomography or ultrasonography of the abdomen can be used to identify CSF-containing cysts that are suggestive of infection.

Treatment of CSF shunt infections is similar to that of VRI. Empiric antimicrobial agents include vancomycin plus an antipseudomonal cephalosporin or carbapenem, based on local resistance patterns. Removal of all components of the infected shunt with placement of an EVD appears to be the most effective treatment, and is strongly encouraged.[75] This method allows for continued CSF diversion and monitoring of CSF parameters. Any remaining foreign bodies (ie, old shunt catheters) present a risk for relapse if they are in continuity with infected CSF, and in those scenarios where components cannot be removed the CSF must be closely monitored. In these scenarios, an antimicrobial-free interval to assess for relapse may be appropriate.

The duration of antimicrobial therapy and the timing of shunt reimplantation have not been studied in a well-controlled prospective trial. According to the Infectious Disease Society of America guidelines on bacterial meningitis,[48] shunt infections due to coagulase-negative staphylococci with normal CSF findings can be reshunted on the third day after removal as long as postremoval cultures remain negative. If the infection is associated with CSF abnormalities, 7 days of antimicrobial therapy is recommended before replacing the shunt as long as repeat cultures are negative. If repeat CSF cultures are positive, antimicrobial treatment is continued until CSF cultures remain negative for 10 consecutive days before a new CSF shunt is placed. For infections with S aureus, fungi, and gram-negative pathogens, 10 to 14 days of antimicrobial therapy with negative cultures is generally recommended.[48] These guidelines are only recommendations, and patients may require longer durations of therapy before reimplantation depending on the clinical situation.

DEEP BRAIN STIMULATOR INFECTIONS

Deep brain stimulators (DBS) are an effective surgical option in the management of movement disorders and chronic pain. However, as with all devices, infection is a known complication. The placement of DBS began in the 1980s and the field has made significant advancements since.[76] The current procedure entails placing an intraparenchymal lead into the brain to deliver electrical impulses that interfere with neural activity at a target site. The lead exits the brain via a burr hole and is tunneled under the scalp, and subcutaneously to the connector site. At the connector site, the lead connects with the extension (often on the head or postauricular) and the extension travels subcutaneously to the internal pulse generator (IPG), most commonly placed in an infraclavicular location (**Fig. 1**). Techniques for this procedure vary considerably, with some institutions placing the lead, extension, and generator in a single phase and others placing the lead initially, followed on a later date by placement of the IPG and extension. Many patients with severe Parkinson disease require bilateral leads, each with their own extension and IPG. New technology now allows a single IPG to power bilateral leads; however, use of this method is not consistent across centers.

All procedures are performed in an operating room under sterile technique. Use of prophylactic antimicrobials is standard practice among neurosurgeons (generally with a first-generation cephalosporin or vancomycin), although duration of postoperative use varies.

Incidence and Risk Factors

Interpretation of the published incidence data is difficult, due to the lack of a standard reportable definition. Some groups may report only infections involving hardware whereas others may report superficial skin infections at the incision sites as well. In the past decade, incidence rates have ranged from 0.62% to 14.3% of patients (**Table 2**). The variability in incidence rates most likely reflects the diversity of the patient population, the variety of surgical techniques available, varying use of antimicrobial prophylaxis, and the definition of infection used. Little is known about the risk factors for development of subsequent infection, due to the lack of a universal reporting system and the small numbers in individual studies. To date, no consistent significant risk factors have been identified in the medical literature; however, age, scalp thickness, underlying comorbid conditions, and operative techniques have all been considered as potential factors.

Infection Types

Infections are commonly found at 1 of 3 sites: the IPG, the connector site, or on the scalp where the lead exits the brain. Early infection (generally considered within 30 days to 6 months of implantation) can be identified by erythema, edema and/or

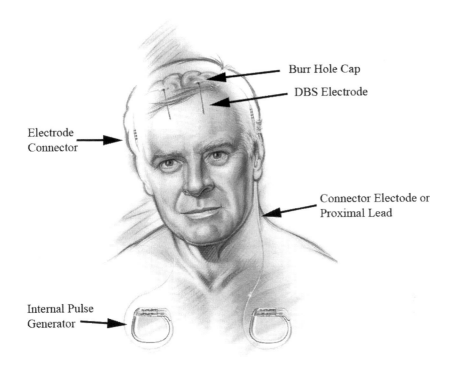

Burr Hole Cap

DBS Electrode

Electrode Connector

Connector Electode or Proximal Lead

Internal Pulse Generator

© Medtronic, Inc. 2008

Fig. 1. A patient with separate bilateral deep brain stimulators (DBS) showing the location of the intracranial lead, extension wire with connector site, and internal pulse generator. (*Courtesy of* Medtronic, Inc; with permission.)

drainage from these sites, or wound dehiscence and hardware exposure. Battery exchanges can also lead to IPG infections potentially years after initial placement. Infrequently patients will present with focal neurologic symptoms and/or seizures caused by an intracranial abscess or cerebritis adjacent to the lead. Erosion at the scalp, connector, and IPG site can occur early, but is the most common presentation of late infection. These patients present with a nonhealing wound over the burr hole or hardware. In the authors' experience, erosion is likely to be a manifestation of underlying infection with a less virulent organism. This scenario results in confusion in the literature, as erosion may be classified as an infectious or a noninfectious complication depending on the institution.

The vast majority of DBS-associated infections are the result of skin flora, with *S aureus, S epidermidis,* and *Propionibacterium acnes* being the most commonly isolated pathogens.[77–79] *Pseudomonas, Enterobacter,* other gram-negatives, and *Mycobacterium fortuitum* have also been isolated.[80,81] Empiric antimicrobial therapy should target skin pathogens including MRSA coverage based on local epidemiology.

Management of Infection

Infections of DBS hardware can lead to serious morbidity due to system removal and resultant poor control of the underlying illness, prolonged hospitalization, prolonged

Table 2
Incidence of deep brain stimulator infections[a]

Study,[Ref.] Year	Country	Years of Study	Patients/Leads	Incidence (n)	Management Details
Doshi,[88] 2011	India	1999–2009	153/298	4.6% (7)	5 required removal of hardware 2 managed with antibiotics alone
Vergani et al,[81] 2010	Italy	1998–2007	141/	5.6% (8)	5 required removal of hardware 3 managed with antibiotics alone
Hu et al,[89] 2010	China	2000–2008	161/259	0.62% (1)	1 required removal of hardware
Fily et al,[79] 2011	France	2006–2008	67/	9.0% (6)	11 required removal of hardware 1 managed with antibiotics alone[b]
Follett et al,[90] 2010	USA	2002–2005	299/598	7.7% (23)	
Gorgulho et al,[77] 2009	USA	1998–2003	139/228	14.3% (20)	12 required removal of hardware 7 managed with antibiotics alone
Seijo et al,[91] 2007	Spain	1998–2005	130/272	1.5% (2)	2 required removal of hardware
Voges et al,[82] 2006	Germany	1996–2003	262/472	5.7% (15)	12 required removal of hardware 3 managed with antibiotics alone
Sillay et al,[78] 2008	USA	1998–2006	420/759	4.5% (19)	19 required removal of hardware
Blomstedt and Hariz,[92] 2002	UK	1993–2002	119/161	3.3% (4)	
Lyons et al,[93] 2004	USA	1997–2002	81/155	6.2% (5)	5 required removal of hardware
Umemura et al,[94] 2003	USA	1998–2002	109/179	3.7% (4)	4 required removal of hardware
Oh et al,[80] 2002	Canada	1993–1999	79/124	15.2% (12)	11 required removal of hardware
Joint et al,[95] 2002	UK	1998–2001	39/79	0	
Beric et al,[96] 2001	USA	1998–2001	86/149	1.2% (1)	
Temel et al,[97] 2004	Netherlands	1996–2002	108/178	3.7% (4)	2 required removal of hardware 2 managed with antibiotics alone

[a] Deep brain stimulation performed for Parkinson disease, essential tremor, chronic pain, dystonia, or other movement disorder.
[b] Management details included cases from other institutions not included in incidence calculation.

antimicrobial use, and repeated surgical procedures. There is currently no consensus on best treatment practices for infections, and management is generally institution specific. The central issue of management revolves around the need to remove infected implants, the timing of removal, and the extent of the removal (partial or complete system removal). The decision to remove a device is not insignificant, due to the need for repeated neurosurgical interventions, the cost of the devices, and the burden placed on the patient.

The majority of management strategies in the medical literature can be classified into 3 groups:

1. Removal of entire system followed by intravenous/oral antimicrobials
2. Brain lead sparing with removal of extension and IPG followed by intravenous/oral antimicrobials
3. Antimicrobials with or without surgical debridement without hardware removal

Gorgulho and colleagues[77] describe 20 device infections, 13 of which were determined to be definite infection based on growth of a microorganism from purulent wound drainage, purulence around the device at time of removal or debridement, and inflammatory changes at the surgical site. Of the 13 patients with definite infections, 12 required complete hardware removal. A brain lead–sparing attempt was made in 2 patients, both of which failed. Seven of the device infections were possible infections based on inflammatory changes at the surgical site and physician-initiated antimicrobial therapy, but negative cultures. All 7 patients were successfully treated with antimicrobial therapy alone.

Voges and colleagues[82] describe their management of 15 device-related skin infections. Skin infections were classified as circumscribed (ie, localized) or "affecting a larger skin area." Five patients received antimicrobial therapy alone, with 2 failures requiring the removal of the entire system. Ten patients underwent immediate debridement and explantation, with 7 patients having the entire system removed.

Sillay and colleagues[78] report on their experience of DBS infections within 6 months of initial implantation. Infections were defined using either clinical (cellulitis directly over hardware or purulent drainage from hardware) or microbiological (positive bacterial culture from a wound swab obtained from hardware or fluid in contact with hardware) evidence. Superficial infections without clinical or microbiological evidence of extension were excluded. An institutional algorithm dictated infection management. If the infection was over the brain lead, demonstrated extensive cellulitis, or multiple drainage sites were present, all hardware was removed and intravenous antimicrobials given. If the patients did not meet these criteria, only the IPG and extension were removed and intravenous antimicrobials were given. Fourteen patients underwent partial removal of the device and 9 went on to complete recovery and subsequent reimplantation. Five patients, however, exhibited evidence of recurrent infection and underwent subsequent total hardware removal. S aureus was identified in 4 of the 5 patients in whom partial hardware removal failed, but was identified in only 2 patients in whom partial hardware removal was successful.

As DBS placement becomes more common, a thoughtful and evidence-based approach to infection is essential. The existing literature is difficult to interpret because of variable follow-up times, as infection can relapse late on. Nevertheless, based on the existing literature and extensive personal observations of one of the authors (W.S.A.), the authors propose the following algorithm. Patients who present with infection at the generator site alone should have an attempt at a brain lead–sparing strategy with only the IPG and extension being removed. Of importance, intracranial infection as a result of brain lead–sparing attempts has not been described in the medical literature. If the connector site has gross evidence of infection, the entire system requires removal. If it does not, the explanted extension at the connector site should be cultured. If positive, the patient has an increased risk of relapse and whole-device removal may be necessary. If it is negative, a trial of antimicrobial therapy is warranted. Two weeks of treatment is generally adequate for a skin and soft-tissue infection.

Patients with infection at the connector site or burr hole are likely to fail any approach short of removal of the entire device, as the intracranial lead itself is nearly always infected. Patients with evidence of intracranial lead infection require a longer course (4–6 weeks) of antimicrobial therapy directed to the CNS. As mentioned earlier, patients with erosion at the burr hole, in the authors' opinion, nearly always have underlying infection as the origin of the erosion, but regardless have infection of the lead. Short-term suppressive antimicrobials can be attempted for those without gross purulence in whom the effect of the system is being studied (eg, dystonia patients in whom a 6-month trial of DBS is necessary to establish efficacy), as nonresponding patients will not require reimplantation. In the long term (years), suppressive therapy is rarely successful. Some centers have attempted flap placement without device removal after debridement of burr hole site erosions, as this is an area of thin skin and mechanical stress.[83,84] Although this may delay presentation of relapse, infection frequently recurs. Also, once a flap has been used, skin coverage options during repeat surgery are limited. Intracranial abscesses occur infrequently but have been described in the literature, and require prompt system removal and prolonged antimicrobial therapy.[79,81]

Unlike ventriculostomy placement, few infection prevention strategies have been evaluated in the medical literature. The authors suggest prophylactic antimicrobials at the time of surgery and 24 hours postoperatively. Agents targeting common skin pathogens (ie, cefazolin or vancomycin) are recommended. Adherence to the guidelines to prevent surgical-site infections is also strongly encouraged.[85]

SUMMARY

CNS device infections remain a challenge to manage because of the risks of repeated operation, inability to perform debridement, and limitations of antimicrobial penetration to the CNS. Nevertheless, CNS devices are becoming more and more commonly used. In addition, devices associated with the peripheral nervous system or which terminate in the epidural space, such as spinal cord stimulators, peripheral nerve stimulators, and intrathecal pumps, are gaining popularity. Data and outcomes of infections associated with these devices are necessary to identify the best preventive and therapeutic management principles. Many lessons from other device-associated and health care–associated infections can be adapted for these devices, including the use of care bundles, impregnated catheters, antimicrobial prophylaxis, and the importance of timely device removal. Additional pharmacokinetic data regarding newer anti-infectives will also aid management decisions.

REFERENCES

1. Dandy WE. An operative procedure for hydrocephalus. Bull Johns Hopkins Hosp 1922;33:189–90.
2. Lozier AP, Sciacca RR, Romagnoli MF, et al. Ventriculostomy-related infections: a critical review of the literature. Neurosurgery 2002;51(1):170–81.
3. Sundbarg G, Nordstrom CH, Soderstrom S. Complications due to prolonged ventricular fluid pressure recording. Br J Neurosurg 1988;2(4):485–95.

4. Holloway KL, Barnes T, Choi S, et al. Ventriculostomy infections: the effect of monitoring duration and catheter exchange in 584 patients. J Neurosurg 1996; 85(3):419–24.
5. Mayhall CG, Archer NH, Lamb VA, et al. Ventriculostomy-related infections. A prospective epidemiologic study. N Engl J Med 1984;310(9):553–9.
6. Hoefnagel D, Dammers R, Ter Laak-Poort MP, et al. Risk factors for infections related to external ventricular drainage. Acta Neurochir (Wien) 2008;150(3): 209–14.
7. Tse T, Cheng K, Wong K, et al. Ventriculostomy and infection: a 4-year-review in a local hospital. Surg Neurol Int 2010;1:47.
8. Chi H, Chang KY, Chang HC, et al. Infections associated with indwelling ventriculostomy catheters in a teaching hospital. Int J Infect Dis 2010;14(3):e216–9.
9. Schade RP, Schinkel J, Visser LG, et al. Bacterial meningitis caused by the use of ventricular or lumbar cerebrospinal fluid catheters. J Neurosurg 2005;102(2): 229–34.
10. Korinek AM, Reina M, Boch AL, et al. Prevention of external ventricular drain-related ventriculitis. Acta Neurochir (Wien) 2005;147(1):39–45.
11. Lo CH, Spelman D, Bailey M, et al. External ventricular drain infections are independent of drain duration: an argument against elective revision. J Neurosurg 2007;106(3):378–83.
12. Lyke KE, Obasanjo OO, Williams MA, et al. Ventriculitis complicating use of intraventricular catheters in adult neurosurgical patients. Clin Infect Dis 2001;33(12): 2028–33.
13. Pfisterer W, Muhlbauer M, Czech T, et al. Early diagnosis of external ventricular drainage infection: results of a prospective study. J Neurol Neurosurg Psychiatry 2003;74(7):929–32.
14. Scheithauer S, Burgel U, Bickenbach J, et al. External ventricular and lumbar drainage-associated meningoventriculitis: prospective analysis of time-dependent infection rates and risk factor analysis. Infection 2010;38(3): 205–9.
15. Scheithauer S, Burgel U, Ryang YM, et al. Prospective surveillance of drain associated meningitis/ventriculitis in a neurosurgery and neurological intensive care unit. J Neurol Neurosurg Psychiatry 2009;80(12): 1381–5.
16. Wong GK, Poon WS, Wai S, et al. Failure of regular external ventricular drain exchange to reduce cerebrospinal fluid infection: result of a randomised controlled trial. J Neurol Neurosurg Psychiatry 2002;73(6):759–61.
17. Winfield JA, Rosenthal P, Kanter RK, et al. Duration of intracranial pressure monitoring does not predict daily risk of infectious complications. Neurosurgery 1993; 33(3):424–30.
18. Arabi Y, Memish ZA, Balkhy HH, et al. Ventriculostomy-associated infections: incidence and risk factors. Am J Infect Control 2005;33(3):137–43.
19. Federico G, Tumbarello M, Spanu T, et al. Risk factors and prognostic indicators of bacterial meningitis in a cohort of 3580 postneurosurgical patients. Scand J Infect Dis 2001;33(7):533–7.
20. Camacho EF, Boszczowski I, Basso M, et al. Infection rate and risk factors associated with infections related to external ventricular drain. Infection 2011;39(1): 47–51.
21. Flibotte JJ, Lee KE, Koroshetz WJ, et al. Continuous antibiotic prophylaxis and cerebral spinal fluid infection in patients with intracranial pressure monitors. Neurocrit Care 2004;1(1):61–8.

22. Horan TC, Andrus M, Dudeck MA. CDC/NHSN surveillance definition of health care-associated infection and criteria for specific types of infections in the acute care setting. Am J Infect Control 2008;36(5): 309–32.

23. Vincent FM. Hypoglycorrhachia after subarachnoid hemorrhage. Neurosurgery 1981;8(1):7–14.

24. Ross D, Rosegay H, Pons V. Differentiation of aseptic and bacterial meningitis in postoperative neurosurgical patients. J Neurosurg 1988;69(5):669–74.

25. Muttaiyah S, Ritchie S, Upton A, et al. Clinical parameters do not predict infection in patients with external ventricular drains: a retrospective observational study of daily cerebrospinal fluid analysis. J Med Microbiol 2008;57(Pt 2): 207–9.

26. Schade RP, Schinkel J, Roelandse FW, et al. Lack of value of routine analysis of cerebrospinal fluid for prediction and diagnosis of external drainage-related bacterial meningitis. J Neurosurg 2006;104(1):101–8.

27. Pfausler B, Beer R, Engelhardt K, et al. Cell index—a new parameter for the early diagnosis of ventriculostomy (external ventricular drainage)-related ventriculitis in patients with intraventricular hemorrhage? Acta Neurochir (Wien) 2004;146(5): 477–81.

28. Martinez R, Gaul C, Buchfelder M, et al. Serum procalcitonin monitoring for differential diagnosis of ventriculitis in adult intensive care patients. Intensive Care Med 2002;28(2):208–10.

29. Berger C, Schwarz S, Schaebitz WR, et al. Serum procalcitonin in cerebral ventriculitis. Crit Care Med 2002;30(8):1778–81.

30. Wong GK, Poon WS, Ip M. Use of ventricular cerebrospinal fluid lactate measurement to diagnose cerebrospinal fluid infection in patients with intraventricular haemorrhage. J Clin Neurosci 2008;15(6):654–5.

31. Deutch S, Dahlberg D, Hedegaard J, et al. Diagnosis of ventricular drainage-related bacterial meningitis by broad-range real-time polymerase chain reaction. Neurosurgery 2007;61(2):306–11.

32. Ibrahim EH, Sherman G, Ward S, et al. The influence of inadequate antimicrobial treatment of bloodstream infections on patient outcomes in the ICU setting. Chest 2000;118(1):146–55.

33. Kumar A, Roberts D, Wood KE, et al. Duration of hypotension before initiation of effective antimicrobial therapy is the critical determinant of survival in human septic shock. Crit Care Med 2006;34(6):1589–96.

34. Marchaim D, Gottesman T, Schwartz O, et al. National multicenter study of predictors and outcomes of bacteremia upon hospital admission caused by Enterobacteriaceae producing extended-spectrum beta-lactamases. Antimicrob Agents Chemother 2010;54(12):5099–104.

35. Pfausler B, Spiss H, Beer R, et al. Treatment of staphylococcal ventriculitis associated with external cerebrospinal fluid drains: a prospective randomized trial of intravenous compared with intraventricular vancomycin therapy. J Neurosurg 2003;98(5):1040–4.

36. Beer R, Engelhardt KW, Pfausler B, et al. Pharmacokinetics of intravenous linezolid in cerebrospinal fluid and plasma in neurointensive care patients with staphylococcal ventriculitis associated with external ventricular drains. Antimicrob Agents Chemother 2007;51(1):379–82.

37. Myrianthefs P, Markantonis SL, Vlachos K, et al. Serum and cerebrospinal fluid concentrations of linezolid in neurosurgical patients. Antimicrob Agents Chemother 2006;50(12):3971–6.

38. Villani P, Regazzi MB, Marubbi F, et al. Cerebrospinal fluid linezolid concentrations in postneurosurgical central nervous system infections. Antimicrob Agents Chemother 2002;46(3):936–7.
39. Rupprecht TA, Pfister HW. Clinical experience with linezolid for the treatment of central nervous system infections. Eur J Neurol 2005;12(7):536–42.
40. Viale P, Pagani L, Cristini F, et al. Linezolid for the treatment of central nervous system infections in neurosurgical patients. Scand J Infect Dis 2002;34(6): 456–9.
41. Boak LM, Li J, Spelman D, et al. Successful treatment and cerebrospinal fluid penetration of oral linezolid in a patient with coagulase-negative *Staphylococcus* ventriculitis. Ann Pharmacother 2006;40(7–8):1451–5.
42. Ntziora F, Falagas ME. Linezolid for the treatment of patients with central nervous system infection. Ann Pharmacother 2007;41(2):296–308.
43. Kethireddy S, Andes D. CNS pharmacokinetics of antifungal agents. Expert Opin Drug Metab Toxicol 2007;3(4):573–81.
44. Tangden T, Enblad P, Ullberg M, et al. Neurosurgical gram-negative bacillary ventriculitis and meningitis: a retrospective study evaluating the efficacy of intraventricular gentamicin therapy in 31 consecutive cases. Clin Infect Dis 2011;52(11): 1310–6.
45. Elvy J, Porter D, Brown E. Treatment of external ventricular drain-associated ventriculitis caused by *Enterococcus faecalis* with intraventricular daptomycin. J Antimicrob Chemother 2008;61(2):461–2.
46. Kim BN, Peleg AY, Lodise TP, et al. Management of meningitis due to antibiotic-resistant *Acinetobacter* species. Lancet Infect Dis 2009;9(4):245–55.
47. Lopez-Alvarez B, Martin-Laez R, Farinas MC, et al. Multidrug-resistant *Acinetobacter baumannii* ventriculitis: successful treatment with intraventricular colistin. Acta Neurochir (Wien) 2009;151(11):1465–72.
48. Tunkel AR, Hartman BJ, Kaplan SL, et al. Practice guidelines for the management of bacterial meningitis. Clin Infect Dis 2004;39(9):1267–84.
49. Mathisen G, Shelub A, Truong J, et al. Coccidioidal meningitis: clinical presentation and management in the fluconazole era. Medicine (Baltimore) 2010;89(5): 251–84.
50. Ziai WC, Lewin JJ 3rd. Improving the role of intraventricular antimicrobial agents in the management of meningitis. Curr Opin Neurol 2009;22(3):277–82.
51. Raad I, Hanna H, Maki D. Intravascular catheter-related infections: advances in diagnosis, prevention, and management. Lancet Infect Dis 2007;7(10):645–57.
52. Mermel LA, Allon M, Bouza E, et al. Clinical practice guidelines for the diagnosis and management of intravascular catheter-related infection: 2009 update by the Infectious Diseases Society of America. Clin Infect Dis 2009;49(1):1–45.
53. Resar R, Pronovost P, Haraden C, et al. Using a bundle approach to improve ventilator care processes and reduce ventilator-associated pneumonia. Jt Comm J Qual Patient Saf 2005;31(5):243–8.
54. Pronovost P, Needham D, Berenholtz S, et al. An intervention to decrease catheter-related bloodstream infections in the ICU. N Engl J Med 2006;355(26): 2725–32.
55. Guerin K, Wagner J, Rains K, et al. Reduction in central line-associated bloodstream infections by implementation of a postinsertion care bundle. Am J Infect Control 2010;38(6):430–3.
56. Leverstein-van Hall MA, Hopmans TE, van der Sprenkel JW, et al. A bundle approach to reduce the incidence of external ventricular and lumbar drain-related infections. J Neurosurg 2010;112(2):345–53.

57. Honda H, Jones JC, Craighead MC, et al. Reducing the incidence of intraventric-
    ular catheter-related ventriculitis in the neurology-neurosurgical intensive care
    unit at a tertiary care center in St Louis, Missouri: an 8-year follow-up study. Infect
    Control Hosp Epidemiol 2010;31(10):1078–81.
58. Sonabend AM, Korenfeld Y, Crisman C, et al. Prevention of ventriculostomy-related
    infections with prophylactic antibiotics and antibiotic-coated external ventricular
    drains: a systematic review. Neurosurgery 2011;68(4):996–1005.
59. Alleyne CH Jr, Hassan M, Zabramski JM. The efficacy and cost of prophylactic
    and periprocedural antibiotics in patients with external ventricular drains. Neuro-
    surgery 2000;47(5):1124–7.
60. Poon WS, Ng S, Wai S. CSF antibiotic prophylaxis for neurosurgical patients with
    ventriculostomy: a randomised study. Acta Neurochir Suppl 1998;71:146–8.
61. Ramos ER, Reitzel R, Jiang Y, et al. Clinical effectiveness and risk of emerging
    resistance associated with prolonged use of antibiotic-impregnated catheters:
    more than 0.5 million catheter days and 7 years of clinical experience. Crit
    Care Med 2011;39(2):245–51.
62. Zabramski JM, Whiting D, Darouiche RO, et al. Efficacy of antimicrobial-
    impregnated external ventricular drain catheters: a prospective, randomized,
    controlled trial. J Neurosurg 2003;98(4):725–30.
63. Muttaiyah S, Ritchie S, John S, et al. Efficacy of antibiotic-impregnated external
    ventricular drain catheters. J Clin Neurosci 2010;17(3):296–8.
64. Tamburrini G, Massimi L, Caldarelli M, et al. Antibiotic impregnated external
    ventricular drainage and third ventriculostomy in the management of hydroceph-
    alus associated with posterior cranial fossa tumours. Acta Neurochir (Wien) 2008;
    150(10):1049–55.
65. Gutierrez-Gonzalez R, Boto GR, Fernandez-Perez C, et al. Protective effect of
    rifampicin and clindamycin impregnated devices against Staphylococcus spp.
    infection after cerebrospinal fluid diversion procedures. BMC Neurol 2010;
    10:93.
66. Abla AA, Zabramski JM, Jahnke HK, et al. Comparison of two antibiotic-
    impregnated ventricular catheters: a prospective sequential series trial. Neuro-
    surgery 2011;68(2):437–42.
67. Harrop JS, Sharan AD, Ratliff J, et al. Impact of a standardized protocol and
    antibiotic-impregnated catheters on ventriculostomy infection rates in cerebro-
    vascular patients. Neurosurgery 2010;67(1):187–91.
68. Stevens EA, Palavecino E, Sherertz RJ, et al. Effects of antibiotic-impregnated
    external ventricular drains on bacterial culture results: an in vitro analysis.
    J Neurosurg 2010;113(1):86–92.
69. Aslam S, Darouiche RO. Prolonged bacterial exposure to minocycline/rifampicin-
    impregnated vascular catheters does not affect antimicrobial activity of catheters.
    J Antimicrob Chemother 2007;60(1):148–51.
70. Wang H, Huang T, Jing J, et al. Effectiveness of different central venous catheters
    for catheter-related infections: a network meta-analysis. J Hosp Infect 2010;76(1):
    1–11.
71. Srinivasan A, Karchmer T, Richards A, et al. A prospective trial of a novel,
    silicone-based, silver-coated Foley catheter for the prevention of nosocomial
    urinary tract infections. Infect Control Hosp Epidemiol 2006;27(1):38–43.
72. Fichtner J, Guresir E, Seifert V, et al. Efficacy of silver-bearing external ventricular
    drainage catheters: a retrospective analysis. J Neurosurg 2010;112(4):840–6.
73. Korinek AM, Fulla-Oller L, Boch AL, et al. Morbidity of ventricular cerebrospinal
    fluid shunt surgery in adults an 8-year study. Neurosurgery 2011;68(4):985–94.

74. Conen A, Walti LN, Merlo A, et al. Characteristics and treatment outcome of cerebrospinal fluid shunt-associated infections in adults: a retrospective analysis over an 11-year period. Clin Infect Dis 2008;47(1):73–82.

75. Whitehead WE, Kestle JR. The treatment of cerebrospinal fluid shunt infections. Results from a practice survey of the American Society of Pediatric Neurosurgeons. Pediatr Neurosurg 2001;35(4):205–10.

76. Benabid AL, Pollak P, Louveau A, et al. Combined (thalamotomy and stimulation) stereotactic surgery of the VIM thalamic nucleus for bilateral Parkinson disease. Appl Neurophysiol 1987;50(1–6):344–6.

77. Gorgulho A, Juillard C, Uslan DZ, et al. Infection following deep brain stimulator implantation performed in the conventional versus magnetic resonance imaging-equipped operating room. J Neurosurg 2009;110(2):239–46.

78. Sillay KA, Larson PS, Starr PA. Deep brain stimulator hardware-related infections: incidence and management in a large series. Neurosurgery 2008;62(2):360–6.

79. Fily F, Haegelen C, Tattevin P, et al. Deep brain stimulation hardware-related infections: a report of 12 cases and review of the literature. Clin Infect Dis 2011;52(8):1020–3.

80. Oh MY, Abosch A, Kim SH, et al. Long-term hardware-related complications of deep brain stimulation. Neurosurgery 2002;50(6):1268–74.

81. Vergani F, Landi A, Pirillo D, et al. Surgical, medical, and hardware adverse events in a series of 141 patients undergoing subthalamic deep brain stimulation for Parkinson disease. World Neurosurg 2010;73(4):338–44.

82. Voges J, Waerzeggers Y, Maarouf M, et al. Deep-brain stimulation: long-term analysis of complications caused by hardware and surgery—experiences from a single centre. J Neurol Neurosurg Psychiatry 2006;77(7):868–72.

83. Lanotte M, Verna G, Panciani PP, et al. Management of skin erosion following deep brain stimulation. Neurosurg Rev 2009;32(1):111–4.

84. Spiotta AM, Bain MD, Deogaonkar M, et al. Methods of scalp revision for deep brain stimulator hardware: case report. Neurosurgery 2008;62(3 Suppl 1):249–50.

85. Anderson DJ, Kaye KS, Classen D, et al. Strategies to prevent surgical site infections in acute care hospitals. Infect Control Hosp Epidemiol 2008;29(Suppl 1): S51–61.

86. Orsi GB, Scorzolini L, Franchi C, et al. Hospital-acquired infection surveillance in a neurosurgical intensive care unit. J Hosp Infect 2006;64(1):23–9.

87. Bota DP, Lefranc F, Vilallobos HR, et al. Ventriculostomy-related infections in critically ill patients: a 6-year experience. J Neurosurg 2005;103(3):468–72.

88. Doshi PK. Long-term surgical and hardware-related complications of deep brain stimulation. Stereotact Funct Neurosurg 2011;89(2):89–95.

89. Hu X, Jiang X, Zhou X, et al. Avoidance and management of surgical and hardware-related complications of deep brain stimulation. Stereotact Funct Neurosurg 2010;88(5):296–303.

90. Follett KA, Weaver FM, Stern M, et al. Pallidal versus subthalamic deep-brain stimulation for Parkinson's disease. N Engl J Med 2010;362(22):2077–91.

91. Seijo FJ, Alvarez-Vega MA, Gutierrez JC, et al. Complications in subthalamic nucleus stimulation surgery for treatment of Parkinson's disease. Review of 272 procedures. Acta Neurochir (Wien) 2007;149(9):867–75.

92. Blomstedt P, Hariz MI. Hardware-related complications of deep brain stimulation: a ten year experience. Acta Neurochir (Wien) 2005;147(10):1061–4.

93. Lyons KE, Wilkinson SB, Overman J, et al. Surgical and hardware complications of subthalamic stimulation: a series of 160 procedures. Neurology 2004;63(4): 612–6.

94. Umemura A, Jaggi JL, Hurtig HI, et al. Deep brain stimulation for movement disorders: morbidity and mortality in 109 patients. J Neurosurg 2003;98(4):779–84.
95. Joint C, Nandi D, Parkin S, et al. Hardware-related problems of deep brain stimulation. Mov Disord 2002;17(Suppl 3):S175–80.
96. Beric A, Kelly PJ, Rezai A, et al. Complications of deep brain stimulation surgery. Stereotact Funct Neurosurg 2001;77(1–4):73–8.
97. Temel Y, Ackermans L, Celik H, et al. Management of hardware infections following deep brain stimulation. Acta Neurochir (Wien) 2004;146(4):355–61.

Breast Implant Infections

Laraine L. Washer, MD[a,b,*], Karol Gutowski, MD[c]

KEYWORDS

• Breast augmentation • Breast implant • Infection

Prosthetic breast implants are used for cosmetic breast enlargement, correction of asymmetries and congenital defects, as well as for breast reconstruction in women who undergo mastectomy for breast cancer or cancer risk reduction. Breast augmentation is the most common cosmetic surgical procedure performed in the United States with 296,203 procedures performed in 2010.[1] Among women who undergo mastectomy, 10% to 20% have a reconstructive procedure and choose prosthetic implants, instead of autologous tissue reconstruction, 80% to 90% of the time.[1,2]

Breast implants may be placed between the pectoralis major muscle and the breast gland (subglandular) or under the muscle (submuscular). In cases of breast reconstruction, the implants are typically placed entirely under the muscle through the mastectomy incision although either the subglandular or the submuscular position may be used for nonreconstructive procedures. For cosmetic purposes, the surgical approach is most commonly through an inframammary or periareolar incision and less commonly using a transaxillary, transareolar, or transumbilical incision. When performed for reconstruction after mastectomy, breast implants can be placed at the time of mastectomy (single-stage) or more commonly at a later time point (two-stage).[3,4]

When using a two-stage approach, a prosthetic tissue expander is placed first under the muscle. Then, after the incision has healed, the expander is filled gradually through a subcutaneous port using weekly saline injections until the proper volume is achieved. At the next stage, the expander is removed and an implant is placed in the expanded pocket. Most commonly for reconstruction, the expander or implant sits in a pocket under the skin and pectoralis major muscle. However, in some types of reconstruction, the expander or implant may be placed under a flap of autologous tissue.

The authors have nothing to disclose.
[a] Division of Infectious Diseases, Department of Internal Medicine, University of Michigan Health System, 3119 Taubman Center, 1500 East Medical Center Drive, Ann Arbor, MI 48109-5378, USA
[b] Department of Infection Control and Epidemiology, University of Michigan Health System, NI8B06 North Ingalls Building, Ann Arbor, MI 48109, USA
[c] Division of Plastic Surgery, University of Chicago Pritzker School of Medicine, Chicago, MC 6035, 5841 South Maryland, Chicago, IL 60637, USA
* Corresponding author. Division of Infectious Diseases, University of Michigan Health System, 3119 Taubman Center, 1500 East Medical Center Drive, Ann Arbor, MI 48109-5378.
E-mail address: laraine@med.umich.edu

Infect Dis Clin N Am 26 (2012) 111–125
doi:10.1016/j.idc.2011.09.003
0891-5520/12/$ – see front matter © 2012 Elsevier Inc. All rights reserved.

id.theclinics.com

The two types of breast implants currently available in the United States are silicone gel and saline implants. Silicone implants contain silicone gel within a silicone polymer shell. Saline implants contain saline within an outer silicone polymer shell. Saline implants are expandable and are filled at the time of insertion by the surgeon. Less common (and currently not available in the United States) are combined saline-silicone gel implants and polyurethane implants. Tissue expanders are similar to saline implants but are made of a thicker shell and have an injection port. Some types of tissue expanders can remain as permanent implants. For purposes of this discussion, unless otherwise specified, the term "implants" will refer to both breast implants and breast tissue expanders because the diagnosis and treatment of associated infections is similar. Acellular dermal matrix (ADM) products (discussed in detail below) may also be used in combination with tissue expander or breast implant surgeries performed for reconstruction.[4–6]

EPIDEMIOLOGY AND COSTS

Reported rates for implant-associated infection after augmentation range from 1.1% to 2.5%.[7–11] Most infections occur in the immediate postoperative period, but infections can also present after many years.[12] Infection rates associated with reconstruction after mastectomy are a magnitude higher, ranging from 1% to 35%.[9,11,13] Hospital-associated costs of surgical site infection (SSI) after breast surgery have been estimated at more than $4000.[14] A lower attributable cost of $574 has been reported when infections are managed completely as outpatient cases.[15] Costs for infectious complications after breast implant surgery are likely higher than for nonimplant breast surgery.

RISK FACTORS

Risk factors for SSI include preoperative, intraoperative, and postoperative factors (**Box 1**). Preoperative factors associated with increased risk of SSI common to all breast surgeries include elevated body mass index, diabetes, smoking, postmenopausal status, prior breast operation, steroid therapy, lymph node resection, preoperative chemotherapy, chest wall radiation, and increased American Surgical Association class. Intraoperative factors associated with increased risk of SSI include duration of the operation, lymph node dissection, higher amount of blood loss, and need for surgical drains. Perioperative antimicrobial prophylaxis and appropriate skin antisepsis are associated with decreased SSI risk. Postoperative factors associated with increased risk of SSI include elevated serum glucose and seroma or hematoma formation.[16] There does not appear to be a difference in infection rates between silicone and saline implants.[17]

Surgical technique is an important contributor to implant infection risk. There may be increased risk of infection with a periareolar or transareolar approach, likely related to potential contamination of the implant by the endogenous flora of the nipple or breast ducts. The surgeon's skill in avoiding the development of hematoma or tissue ischemia is another important way to decrease the risk of infection. The use of surgical drains has been associated with as much as a fivefold risk of breast implant infection in some studies.[7] However, a single-center review of 2446 procedures in which tissue expanders were exchanged for permanent breast implants found no difference in the rate of infection necessitating implant removal among those who had drains placed compared with those who did not.[18]

Infection rates among reconstruction surgeries are significantly higher than primary breast augmentation procedures. Among women undergoing breast reconstruction,

Box 1
Potential risk factors for breast implant infection
Elevated body mass index
Diabetes
Smoking
Postmenopausal
Prior breast operation
Steroid therapy
American Surgical Association class
Drain placement
Radiation therapy
Chemotherapy
Longer operative times
Lymph node dissection
Immediate implant after mastectomy
Breast size larger than C cup
Repeated implant placement
Seroma or hematoma formation

additional factors associated with infection include receipt of radiation therapy or adjuvant chemotherapy, longer operative times with two surgical teams, and lymph node dissection.[19] Immediate placement of an implant after mastectomy also increases infection risk compared with delayed implant placement.[12] A two-stage procedure is postulated to allow time for endogenous breast flora to be eliminated from the surgical bed. Risk factors for infection among patients undergoing tissue-expander breast reconstruction include breast size larger than C cup, previous chest wall radiation, and repeated implant placement.[20] In one study of women undergoing mastectomy and immediate breast reconstruction, the highest overall rate of SSI was among those receiving adjuvant chemotherapy (44%) compared with those getting neoadjuvant chemotherapy (23%) or no chemotherapy (25%).[19]

Acellular dermal matrix (ADM) is comprised of dermal allograft biomaterial in which all the cellular elements have been removed. By providing breast implant coverage inside the breast pocket, use of ADM allows for easier immediate breast reconstruction following mastectomy. Early versions of ADM products were derived from human cadaver dermis that was treated to remove all cadaver cells and potential pathogens, leaving behind an acellular connective tissue matrix. Over time, the patient's own cells repopulate the matrix and allow for tissue in-growth and full tissue integration. Unfortunately, in some cases, the ADM does not integrate with the patient's tissue and may be associated with infection, impaired healing, or extrusion of the prosthesis. Newer versions of these products include processing modifications to allow for better tissue in-growth, the use of nonhuman tissue (commonly bovine or porcine sources), and the use of nondermal tissues (intestinal submucosa, pericardium).

Currently, there are many types, brands, and variations of ADMs and ADM-like products (both of human and animal sources), each with its own unique characteristics and ability for tissue integration. Because of these variables, specific infection and complication rates associated with ADM use are not well defined, but the use of ADM-like materials is associated with increased rates of SSI in some studies. A meta-analysis of 12 studies including 789 breasts identified an infection rate of 5.6% with use of ADM.[21] Antony and colleagues[22] reported that use of ADM was associated with increased complications of seroma and reconstructive failure, some of which were due to infection. A separate report of 470 patients undergoing immediate reconstruction after mastectomy found that use of ADM was associated with an increase in infections requiring removal of the prosthesis (4.2%) compared with reconstruction without use of ADM (2.4%).[23] In contrast, Salzberg and colleagues[24] found no difference in overall complication rate (including infection) with ADM use in immediate breast reconstruction.

Use of ADM has been associated with a phenomenon of "red breast syndrome" that often presents as painless blanching erythema of the inferior breast overlying the ADM site. Although red breast syndrome is not completely understood, it is not thought to be infectious in origin. Some theorize that it may be due to dependent erythema, interruption of lymphatic flow, generalized histamine release, or hyperemia of the overlying skin due to dilation of the cutaneous vascular network as the graft material develops vascular ingrowth. The red breast syndrome after ADM placement is commonly confused for a breast cellulitis or infection but is self-limited and resolves spontaneously in a period of weeks to months.[21]

PATHOGENESIS AND MICROBIOLOGY

The breast is not sterile and endogenous skin flora colonizing the nipple can be transmitted to deeper breast tissue via breast ducts or during a surgical procedure resulting in infection. Coagulase negative staphylococci can be isolated from the breast in more than half of women at the time of breast augmentation or reduction. Other skin flora frequently isolated from the breast includes diphtheroids, lactobacilli, bacillus species, beta hemolytic streptococci, and *Propionibacterium acnes*.[25] Contamination of the breast prosthesis with these endogenous flora during surgery is responsible for most implant infections. Other less common mechanisms of breast implant infections include contamination of the implant or saline from the surgical environment, from skin-penetrating trauma, including body piercings, and hematogenous contamination of the implant from infection at a distant site.[3]

Once colonized, implants have a high risk for symptomatic infection due to formation of biofilms.[26] Biofilms are complex structures that form when bacteria adhere to artificial surfaces. Biofilms are composed of both bacteria and an extracellular matrix of polymeric material produced by bacteria. Because of altered bacterial metabolism and the extracellular matrix, bacteria embedded in biofilms are often resistant to killing by antimicrobials despite in vitro susceptibility.[27] Once established, biofilms are often impossible to eradicate without removal of the associated foreign body.[28]

Up to two-thirds of infections occur within the first month after implant surgery.[12] On average, saline breast implant infections occur earlier than silicone implant infections.[17] Patients with early onset infections typically present with breast pain, swelling, and erythema, with or without fever. Purulent drainage may be present at the incision. These symptoms can reflect simple cellulitis or infection of the actual implant. Ultrasound will sometimes reveal fluid surrounding the breast implant. Leukocytosis may be present, but it is not sensitive or specific.[3]

Gram-positive organisms (*Staphylococcus aureus*, streptococci, coagulase negative staphylococcus, *Propionibacterium* spp) are the usual pathogens associated with early postimplant infections. In a study of acute postoperative breast implant infections at a single Texas hospital, 67% of breast implant infections were due to *S aureus* with 68% of *S aureus* infections being methicillin-resistant *S aureus* (MRSA). In the same study, gram-negative bacteria were associated with just 6% of infections; cultures were sterile in 26%.[29]

In addition to local signs of infection, patients with breast implants may present with toxic shock syndrome (TSS) if the infection is due to toxin-producing *S aureus* (**Box 2**) or streptococcus (**Box 3**).[30,31] Patients with TSS can present immediately after surgery (within 12–24 hours), although the median time to presentation is 4 days.[32] TSS is associated with fever, hypotension, and sepsis. In addition, diffuse rash, nausea, vomiting, diarrhea, and multiorgan system failure with elevated creatinine, abnormal liver function tests, or acute respiratory distress syndrome may be present.[33] Overt signs of infection may not be present at the surgical site; therefore, when patients present with sepsis soon after implant placement, clinicians must have a high suspicion for breast implant infection. In cases of implant associated TSS, prompt removal of the prosthesis is imperative to patient survival.

Subacute infections may present several months postoperatively with symptoms such as breast pain or drainage, prolonged wound healing, extrusion or movement of the implant, or, simply, general malaise. Subacute infections are most commonly due to coagulase negative staphylococcus and *Propionibacterium* spp.

Box 2
TSS clinical case definition

Fever

Temperature >38.9°C

Hypotension

Systolic blood pressure (BP) ≤90 mmHg or

Orthostatic decrease in diastolic BP ≥15 mmHg

Rash—diffuse macular erythroderma

Desquamation—especially involving palms and soles occurring 1–2 weeks after illness

Multisystem involvement—three or more of following systems

Gastrointestinal: vomiting or diarrhea

Musculoskeletal: myalgia or creatine phosphokinase elevation >2 times normal

Mucous membranes: hyperemia of vaginal, oropharyngeal, conjunctival mucosa

Renal: serum urea nitrogen or serum creatinine ≥2 times normal

Hepatic: bilirubin or transaminase ≥2 times normal

Hematologic: platelets <100,000/uL

Central nervous system: alterations in consciousness or disorientation without focal neurologic signs (in absence of fever and hypotension)

Negative results—if obtained

Blood, throat, or cerebrospinal fluid cultures for another pathogen (blood cultures may be positive for *S aureus*.)

Serologic tests for Rocky Mountain spotted fever, leptospirosis, or measles

Adapted from Centers for Disease Control and Prevention. Case definitions for infectious conditions under public health surveillance. MMWR Recomm Rep 1997;46(RR-10):1–55.

Box 3
Streptococcal TSS case definition

Hypotension

Systolic blood pressure ≤90 mmHg

Multiorgan involvement with two or more of the following:

Renal impairment: creatinine ≥2 mg/dL or ≥2 × baseline

Coagulopathy: platelets ≤100,000/mm³ or DIC

Liver involvement: bilirubin or transaminases ≥2 × normal or ≥2 × baseline

Acute respiratory distress syndrome

Generalized erythematous macular rash that may desquamate

Soft tissue necrosis

Laboratory criteria for diagnosis

Isolation of Group A *Streptococcus*

Abbreviation: DIC, disseminated intravascular coagulation.

Adapted from Centers for Disease Control and Prevention. Case definitions for infectious conditions under public health surveillance. MMWR Recomm Rep 1997;46(RR-10):1–55.

Late infections (months to years after surgery) are uncommon and may present only with vague breast pain with or without inflammatory skin changes. Infections of breast implants have been described following infections at distant sites implicating secondary, hematogenous seeding of the implant as a pathogenic mechanism. Late infections may be associated with gram-positive or gram-negative organisms if related to bacteremia. Several examples are reported, including a periprosthetic breast abscess with *Streptococcus pyogenes* after scarlet fever,[34] *Clostridium perfringens* breast implant infection after dental treatment,[35] and *Klebsiella pneumoniae* breast implant infection after *K pneumoniae* bacteremia.[36]

Late infections have also occurred in the setting of outbreaks due to poor infection-control practices. One notable outbreak involved four patients who presented with *Serratia marcescens*–associated implant infection a median of 66 days (range 13–161) postoperatively. *S marcescens* was cultured from a bag of saline used for expansion in the surgeon's office. The infections were likely related to the repeated use of an individual saline bag that was extrinsically contaminated due to poor hand hygiene and breaks in aseptic technique at the time of implant expansion.[37]

Nontuberculous mycobacterial (NTM) implant infections are being reported with increasing frequency. Clinically, NTM infections may present as acute, subacute, or late-onset infections and they have been reported both as sporadic cases and outbreaks. A review of 10 patients with NTM breast implant infection from two Canadian cities reported that clinical presentation of NTM breast infection was similar to non–mycobacterial breast implant infection with median time to symptom onset of 4.5 weeks. Four of ten patients had bilateral breast implant infection.[38] When cultures for routine bacterial pathogens are negative, NTM infection should be considered and acid-fast bacterial cultures obtained.

Mycobacterium fortuitum[38–41] is the most common NTM species associated with breast implant infection, but multiple other species of NTM have been described. These include *M avium*,[42,43] *M abscessus*,[44,45] *M conceptionense*,[46] *M thermoreistible*[47] and *M chelonae*.[40,48] One outbreak of NTM wound infections associated with breast augmentation was attributed to contaminated gentian violet skin-marking solution.[49] Another noteworthy outbreak of *M jacuzzii* infection involved 10 women with breast implants. It was linked to colonization of human skin with *M jacuzzii* when molecular typing of cultured surgical wound isolates matched isolates from the surgeon's body hair and home whirlpool.[50]

Other uncommon organisms are reported including *Streptomyces*,[51] *Pasteurella multicida*,[52] *Brucella*[53] and *Granulicatella adiacens*.[54] Fungal infections are rare causes of breast implant infections but infection due to *Trichosporon*,[55] *Aspergillus flavus*,[56] and *Candida albicans*[57] are all described.

Fibrosis surrounding breast implants causing capsular contracture is associated with unwanted cosmetic appearance, firmness of the breast, breast distortion, and pain. It has been postulated that contracture is related to chronic infection with coagulase-negative staphylococcus and skin organisms are commonly cultured from breast implants removed for capsular contracture.

Among 22 breast implants removed with capsular fibrosis, 41% grew skin organisms including coagulase-negative staphylococcus, *Propionibacterium acnes*, or both.[58] Among 27 implants removed at the Mayo Clinic for capsular contracture, 9 (33%) had *Propionibacterium* spp, coagulase-negative staphylococcus, or *Corynebacterium* spp isolated, whereas only 1 of 18 (5%) that were removed for reasons other than capsular contracture demonstrated growth of skin organisms.[59] An in vivo model of augmentation mammoplasty in pigs found that implants inoculated with coagulase-negative *Staphylococcus* had biofilm formation and subsequent capsular contracture, whereas contracture did not occur in implants that were not inoculated with coagulase-negative *Staphylococcus*.[60] Carlesimo and colleagues[61] described a regimen of preoperative, intraoperative, and postoperative antimicrobials to prevent capsular contracture among 67 patients with a 2 to 9 year follow-up period. They found no patients had advanced capsular contracture or had need for prosthesis removal. Although this protocol has potential in reducing biofilm-associated infections and capsular contracture around breast implants, the small patient group and relatively short follow-up interval does not allow for a clinical recommendation based on a high level of evidence.

DIAGNOSIS

Differentiation among red breast syndrome, cellulitis, superficial surgical site infection, and implant (deep) infection is essential for management (**Fig. 1**). Any draining fluid should be cultured. However, the swab technique of draining fluid for culture is generally not useful due to skin contaminants. If present, ultrasound imaging and guided aspiration of periprosthetic fluid collections is the preferred approach. The absence of a fluid collection on ultrasound does not rule out implant infection, so lack of clinical improvement after an appropriate period of antimicrobial treatment may necessitate implant removal.

At the time of surgical device removal, the implant should be cultured. Specimens should be sent for standard aerobic and anaerobic bacteria, fungal, and mycobacterial cultures. Tissue, if removed, should be examined histopathologically.[3] Among patients with sepsis, blood cultures should be obtained to assess for concomitant bacteremia. In cases of late-onset breast swelling and seroma formation in the breast pocket that do not present like typical breast infections, cytology and other specialized immunohistochemistry testing of the periprosthetic fluid is indicated to evaluate for malignancy such as breast carcinoma or anaplastic, large cell lymphoma, a rare condition recently described in association with breast implants.[62]

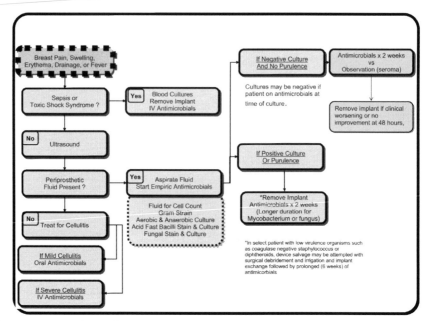

Fig. 1. Breast implant infection: diagnosis and management.

MANAGEMENT

There are no randomized, controlled trials of breast implant infection that directly compare implant removal with salvage. Historically, management of breast implant infection has included systemic antimicrobial therapy and implant removal in most cases. Antimicrobial therapy should be started while awaiting culture results (see **Fig. 1**). There are no established guidelines for empiric antimicrobial therapy for breast implant infections. However, because of the high incidence of beta-lactam–resistant pathogens, including MRSA and methicillin-resistant, coagulase-negative *Staphylococcus*, vancomycin should be a part of initial empiric therapy.[29] Additional coverage for gram-negative bacteria with broad spectrum cephalosporins or extended spectrum penicillins is reasonable pending culture results. Antimicrobials should be tailored to target pathogens identified on culture. After implant removal, systemic antimicrobials should be continued for 10 to 14 days for standard bacterial infections and several months for mycobacterial infections.[38,63] Macadam and colleagues[38] reported a median of 22 weeks of antimicrobial therapy for mycobacterial breast-implant infections with regimens varying based on the species of NTM.

Reimplantation may be considered after treatment and a device-free period, assuming there is complete resolution of residual infection. Reimplantation is often delayed by 3 to 6 months to assure infection is resolved, but there are no trials identifying optimal timing.[3] Halvorson and colleagues[64] evaluated outcomes of infected breast-tissue expanders. Among nine patients who underwent secondary implant placement, eight were successful and one patient developed recurrent infection requiring explantation.

Implant removal is often necessary for cure and should be considered early in the case of sepsis or lack of response to antimicrobial therapy. However, because implant removal is costly and often devastating to the patient, treatment with antimicrobials without implant removal is occasionally attempted (especially if cellulitis alone is present) and may be a valid approach for a subset of patients.[65] If symptoms persist despite treatment, surgery to explore and irrigate the pocket and obtain cultures should be performed. Although removal of the implant at this point is the most conservative approach, some investigators have reported successful implant salvage with a protocol of 6 weeks of systemic antimicrobials combined with lavage of the pocket and exchange of the implant[66] or with implant salvage with use of an implant sizer and negative-pressure wound management.[67] Chun and Schulman[6] report successful salvage of nine infected implants in eight consecutive patients who had undergone mastectomy with immediate tissue expander or implant reconstruction. All eight patients were treated with intravenous antimicrobials, drainage of periprosthetic fluid, debridement of the infected pocket, and device exchange.[6] Courtiss and colleagues[13] reported that, among 29 patients, 13 (45%) with a periprosthetic infection with drainage, erythema, swelling, and/or pain were treated successfully with antimicrobials and wound drainage. Spear and colleagues[65] reported a 76.9% implant salvage rate among 24 patients with 26 implants with infection or threatened or actual prosthesis exposure with an algorithmic approach, including aggressive interventions of antimicrobials, debridement, curettage, pulse lavage, capsulectomy, device exchange, and primary closure or flap coverage. Risk factors for failed device salvage included infection with atypical pathogens (NTM, fungi), gram-negative rods, or MRSA. Recurrent device infection was strongly associated with history of radiotherapy or *S aureus* infection.[68]

Although salvage of an obviously infected breast implant or tissue expander is possible in selected patients using these aggressive protocols, the risks of extended courses of intravenous antimicrobials, central venous access, hospitalization, and reoperation for treatment failure should be carefully considered and candidly discussed. Patients with poor soft-tissue coverage of the breast, wound healing problems, and the need to progress to the next stage of breast cancer treatment may be better served by removal of the prosthesis and replacement in 3 to 6 months.

PREVENTION

The fundamentals of general SSI prevention also apply to breast surgery and careful attention to preoperative, intraoperative, and postoperative practices can decrease risk. Because preoperative showering with antiseptic or antibacterial soaps results in decreased bacterial counts on skin, this practice is recommended by the US Centers for Disease Control and Prevention but has not clearly been associated with decreased SSI rates. Preparation of the incision site should include an aseptically applied skin-preparation agents such as an iodophor, alcohol-containing product or chlorhexidine gluconate. Alcohol can be used as part of the skin-preparation regimen but should not be used as a single agent. All members of the surgical team should perform careful preoperative hand and forearm skin antisepsis and should follow proper surgical attire standards, including avoiding long or artificial nails and jewelry. Standards for operating room ventilation should be followed and in-and-out traffic should be kept to a minimum, especially at the time of implant placement.[69,70]

Preoperative prophylactic antimicrobials are associated with decreased risk of postoperative wound infections in breast surgery and are recommended before breast implant surgeries.[71,72] In a large survey of 39,455 patients undergoing breast augmentation, receipt of prophylactic systemic antimicrobials before surgical incision was associated with a significant decreased infection rate (0.42% with prophylaxis compared with 0.87% without prophylaxis).[73] Antimicrobials selection, timing of administration in relationship to incision, weight-based dosing, and redosing for prolonged operative duration are all important components of surgical prophylaxis.[74]

Cefazolin is generally recommended to provide coverage against common skin flora. Alternatives for patients with severe penicillin allergy include vancomycin or clindamycin. Antimicrobials should be administered within 30 minutes before surgical incision to insure that adequate tissue concentration is achieved at the time of incision. If vancomycin is used, it should be administered over 90 minutes beginning 2 hours before incision to insure adequate tissue concentrations at the time of surgery.[75,76] Higher doses of drug may be indicated for obese patients. Olsen and colleagues[16] found that receiving a suboptimal dose of cefazolin among patients with a body mass index greater than 30 was associated with increased risk of SSI. Cefazolin 1 g is recommended for normal-weight patients, but a 2 g dose should be considered for patients greater than 80 to 100 kg.[74] If the procedure is less than 3 to 4 hours in length, a single dose of antimicrobial is adequate to provide good tissue levels for the entire operation. For surgeries lasting 4 hours or longer, redosing of drugs with shorter half-lives, such as cefazolin, should be considered.[74,76]

Although practice among plastic surgeons reveals that preoperative antimicrobial use is nearly universal (98%), there is variation among postoperative use. In a 2009 survey of plastic surgeons, 72% of surgeons opted for postoperative antimicrobials.[77] However, available data suggest that prolonged durations of postoperative antimicrobials do not impact infection risk and extended use may be associated with complications (nausea, vomiting, diarrhea, rash) in more than 5% of breast surgery patients.[78] A retrospective analysis of 1628 primary augmentation mammoplasties found that a single dose of antimicrobial is adequate for prophylaxis in breast augmentation surgery and that longer durations of use did not result in reduced rates of either superficial or periprosthetic infection.[79] In this study, a single preincision dose of antimicrobials was associated with a 0.8% superficial wound infection rate and a 0% periprosthetic infection rate, whereas a single preincision dose followed by 5 days of oral antibiotics was associated with a 1.1% superficial wound infection rate and a 0.65% periprosthetic infection rate.

Topical antimicrobials and antiseptics used for irrigation of the surgical pocket at the time of breast augmentation have been proposed as additional strategies to reduce infection risk but there are no randomized trials to support or refute this practice. A systematic review examining the efficacy of povidone-iodine irrigation to prevent SSI concluded that 10 of 15 studies found povidone iodine irrigation was more effective at preventing SSI when compared with interventions of saline, water, or no intervention; however, none of these studies focused on breast implant surgeries.[80] The US Food and Drug Administration banned the use of povidone iodine for saline breast implant surgeries in 2001 owing to concern for higher rates of implant deflation with use of povidone iodine irrigation.[81]

A retrospective study of 3000 implant surgeries found that local irrigation of the implant pocket with cefuroxime and gentamicin plus povidone iodine was associated with a fourfold decreased incidence of infections when compared with povidone iodine irrigation alone.[7] Another retrospective study of 436 patients reported that adding cephalothin to the irrigation of the breast implant pocket was associated with a significant decrease in SSI rates (6.7%) compared with SSI rates (12.8%) with use of normal saline irrigation.[82] The generalizability of these results is limited both by the retrospective design and a high baseline infection rate.

Others have suggested that the use of topical antiinfective agents for irrigation of the breast implant pocket at the time of surgery has been associated with decreased rates of capsular contracture. Adams and colleagues reported that breast pocket irrigation with a combination of cefazolin, gentamicin, bacitracin, and normal saline was associated with a lower than expected rate of capsular contracture (1.8% primary breast augmentation and 9.5% in breast reconstruction).[83] A prospective, randomized, double-blind study evaluated the effect of various local antimicrobial agents, including, intraprosthetic cephalothin with or without povidone iodine, povidone iodine alone, or antibiotic-steroid foam were each associated with a sevenfold (85%) reduction in early-onset capsular contracture compared with a control arm without local antimicrobial or antiseptic irrigation.[84] Antimicrobial impregnation of the breast tissue expander sleeve has been suggested as a possible approach to decrease infection risk but there are no clinical data to support efficacy.[85]

Strict aseptic technique when filling tissue expanders with saline in the outpatient setting should be followed. This includes proper hand hygiene; use of skin antisepsis before accessing the subcutaneous port; use of sterile saline in a single-patient, single-use manner; and maintenance of a closed system when filling the tissue expander with saline.

SUMMARY

Breast implant surgeries for augmentation and reconstruction are commonly performed. Infection occurs in 1.1% to 2.5% of primary augmentation cases and up to 35% of reconstruction cases. Early infections most commonly result from gram-positive bacteria, including streptococcus and S aureus. Delayed infections may be associated with more indolent bacteria such as coagulase negative staphylococcus, due to secondary infection of the implant because of hematogenous infection or, rarely, as a result of atypical infectious agents, including mycobacterium and fungus. Removal of the implant is frequently required but salvage can be attempted in carefully selected situations.

REFERENCES

1. American Society of Plastic Surgeons Report of the 2010 Plastic Surgery Statistics. 2010. Available at: http://www.plasticsurgery.org/News-and-Resources/Statistics.html. Accessed May 3, 2011.
2. Alderman A, Wei Y, Birkmeyer J. Use of breast reconstruction after mastectomy following the Women's Health and Cancer Rights Act. JAMA 2006;295(4):387–8.
3. Pittet B, Montandon D, Pittet D. Infection in breast implants. Lancet Infect Dis 2005;5:94–106.
4. Cordeiro P. Breast reconstruction after surgery for breast cancer. N Engl J Med 2008;359(15):1590–601.
5. FDA Breast Implant Consumer Handbook 2004. Available at: http://www.fda.gov/MedicalDevices/ProductsandMedicalProcedures/ImplantsandProsthetics/Breastimplants/ucm064106.htm. Accessed May 18, 2011.
6. Chun J, Schulman M. The infected breast prosthesis after mastectomy reconstruction: successful salvage of nine implants in eight consecutive patients. Plast Reconstr Surg 2007;120(3):581–9.
7. Araco A, Gravante G, Araco F, et al. Infections of breast implants in aesthetic breast augmentations: a single-center review of 3002 patients. Aesthetic Plast Surg 2007;31(4):325–9.
8. Hvilsom G, Holmich L, Henriksen T, et al. Local complications after cosmetic breast augmentation: results from the Danish Registry for Plastic Surgery of the Breast. Plast Surg Nurs 2010;30(3):172–9.

9. Alderman A, Wilkins E, Kim H, et al. Complications in postmastectomy breast reconstruction: two-year results of the Michigan Breast Reconstruction Outcome Study. Plast Reconstr Surg 2002;109:2265–74.

10. Kjoller K, Holmich L, Jacobsen P, et al. Epidemiological investigation of local complications after cosmetic breast implant surgery in Denmark. Ann Plast Surg 2004;48(3):229–37.

11. Gabriel S, Woods J, O'Fallon W, et al. Complications leading to surgery after breast implantation. N Engl J Med 1997;336(10):677–82.

12. de Cholnoky T. Augmentation mammaplasty. Survey of complications in 10.941 patients by 265 surgeons. Plast Reconstr Surg 1970;45(6):573–7.

13. Courtiss E, Goldwyn R, Anastasi G. The fate of breast implants with infection around them. Plast Reconstr Surg 1979;63(6):812–6.

14. Olsen M, Chu-Ongsakul S, Brandt K, et al. Hospital-associated costs due to surgical site infection after breast surgery. Arch Surg 2008;143(1):53–60.

15. Reilly J, Twaddle S, McIntosh J, et al. An economic analysis of surgical wound infection. J Hosp Infect 2001;49:245–9.

16. Olsen M, Lefta M, Dietz J, et al. Risk factors for surgical site infection after major breast operation. J Am Coll Surg 2008;207:326–35.

17. Basile A, Basile F, Basile A. Late infection following breast augmentation with textured silicone gel-filled implants. Aesthet Surg J 2005;25(3):249–54.

18. McCarthy C, Disa J, Pusic A, et al. The effect of closed-suction drains on the incidence of local wound complications following tissue expander/implant reconstruction: a cohort study. Plast Reconstr Surg 2008;119(7):2018–22.

19. Peled A, Itakura K, Foster R, et al. Impact of chemotherapy on postoperative complications after mastectomy and immediate breast reconstruction. Arch Surg 2010;145(9):880–5.

20. Francis S, Ruberg R, Stevenson K, et al. Independent risk factors for infection in tissue expander breast reconstruction. Plast Reconstr Surg 2009;124:1790–6.

21. Newman M, Swartz K, Samson M, et al. The true incidence of near-term postoperative complications in prosthetic breast reconstruction utilizing human acellular dermal matrices: a meta-analysis. Aesthetic Plast Surg 2011;35(1):100–6.

22. Antony A, McCarthy C, Cordeiro P, et al. Acellular human dermis implantation in 153 immediate two-stage tissue expander breast reconstructions: determining the incidence and significant predictors of complications. Plast Reconstr Surg 2010;125:1606–24.

23. Liu A, Kao H, Reish R, et al. Post-operative complications in prosthesis-based breast reconstruction using acellular dermal matrix. Plast Reconstr Surg 2011; 127(5):1755–62.

24. Salzberg C, Ashikari A, Koch R, et al. An 8-year experience of direct-to-implant immediate breast reconstruction using human acellular dermal matrix (AlloDerm). Plast Reconstr Surg 2011;127(2):514–24.

25. Thornton J, Argenta L, McClatchey K, et al. Studies on the endogenous flora of the human breast. Ann Plast Surg 1988;20(1):39–42.

26. Dougherty S. Pathobiology of infection in prosthetic devices. Rev Infect Dis 1988; 10(6):1102–17.

27. Costerton J, Stewart P, Greenberg E. Bacterial biofilms: a common cause of persistent infections. Science 1999;284:1318–21.

28. Costerton J, Montanaro L, Arciola C. Biofilm in implant infections: its production and regulation. Int J Artif Organs 2005;28(11):1062–8.

29. Feldman E, Kontoyiannis D, Sharabi S, et al. Breast implant infections: is cefazolin enough? Plast Reconstr Surg 2010;126:779–85.

30. Kohannim O, Rubin Z, Taylor M. Saline breast implant fluid collection and reactive arthritis in a patient with streptococcal toxic shock syndrome. J Clin Rheumatol 2011;17(2):89–91.
31. Tobin G, Shaw R, Goodpasture H. Toxic shock syndrome following breast and nasal surgery. Plast Reconstr Surg 1987;80(1):111–4.
32. Holm C, Muhlbauer W. Toxic shock syndrome in plastic surgery patients: case report and review of the literature. Aesthetic Plast Surg 1998;22:180–4.
33. Mandell G, Bennett J, Dolin R, editors. 6th edition, Mandell, Douglas, and Bennett's principles and practice of infectious diseases, vol. 2. Philadelphia: Elsevier, Churcill, Livingstone; 2005.
34. Persichetti P, Langella M, Marangi G, et al. Periprosthetic breast abscess caused by *Streptococcus pyogenes* after scarlet fever. Ann Plast Surg 2008;60(1):21–3.
35. Hunter J, Padilla M, Cooper-Vastola S. Late *Clostridium perfringens* breast implant infection after dental treatment. Ann Plast Surg 1996;36(3):309–12.
36. Bernardi C, Saccomanno F. Late *Klebsiella pneumoniae* infection following breast augmentation: case report. Aesthetic Plast Surg 1998;22:222–4.
37. Pegues D, Shireley L, Riddle C, et al. *Serratia marcescens* surgical wound infection following breast reconstruction. Am J Med 1991;91:173S–8S.
38. Macadam S, Mehling B, Fanning A, et al. Nontuberculous mycobacterial breast implant infections. Plast Reconstr Surg 2007;119(1):337–44.
39. Vinh D, Rendina A, Turner R, et al. Breast implant infection with *Mycobacterium fortuitum* group: report of case and review. J Infect 2005;52:e63–7.
40. Boettcher A, Bengston B, Farber S, et al. Breast infections with atypical mycobacteria following reduction mammaplasty. Aesthet Surg J 2010;30(4):542–8.
41. Haiavy J, Tobin H. *Mycobacterium fortuitum* infection in prosthetic breast implants. Plast Reconstr Surg 2002;109(6):2124–8.
42. Pereira L, Sterodimas A. Autologous fat transplantation and delayed silicone implant insertion in a case of *Mycobacterium avium* breast infection. Aesthetic Plast Surg 2010;34(1):1–4.
43. Wirth G, Brenner K, Sundine M. Delayed silicone breast implant infection with *Mycobacterium avium*-intracellulare. Aesthet Surg J 2007;27(2):167–71.
44. Feldman E, Ellsworth W, Yuksel E, et al. *Mycobacterium abscessus* infection after breast augmentation: a case of contaminated implants? J Plast Reconstr Aesthet Surg 2009;62(9):e330–2.
45. Jackowe D, Murariu D, Parsa N, et al. Chronic fistulas after breast augmentation secondary to *Mycobacterium abscessus*. Plast Reconstr Surg 2010;126(1):38e–9e.
46. Thibeaut S, Levy PY, Pelletier ML, et al. *Mycobacterium conceptionense* after breast implant infection, France. Emerg Infect Dis 2010;16(7):1180–1.
47. Wolfe J, Moore D. Isolation of *Mycobacterium thermoresistibile* following augmentation mammaplasty. J Clin Microbiol 1992;30:1036–8.
48. Padoveze MF, Fortaleza CM, Freire M, et al. Outbreak of surgical infection caused by non-tuberculous mycobacteria in breast implants in Brazil. J Hosp Infect 2007;67(2):161–7.
49. Safranek T, Jarvis W, Carson L, et al. *Mycobacterium chelonae* wound infection after plastic surgery employing contaminated gentian violet skin-marking solution. N Engl J Med 1987;171(4):197–201.
50. Rahav G, Pitlik S, Amitai Z, et al. An outbreak of *Mycobacterium jacuzzii* infection following insertion of breast implants. Clin Infect Dis 2006;43:823–30.
51. Manteca A, Palaez A, del Mar Garcia-Suarex M, et al. A rare case of silicone mammary implant infection by *Streptomyces* spp. in a patient with breast

reconstruction after mastectomy: taxonomic characterization using molecular techniques. Diagn Microbiol Infect Dis 2009;63(4):390–3.

52. Mathieu D, Rodriguez H, Jacobs F. Breast prosthesis infected by *Pasteurella multocida*. Acta Clin Belg 2008;63(5):351.

53. De B, Stauffer L, Koylass M, et al. Novel *Brucella* strain (BO1) associated with a prosthetic breast implant infection. J Clin Microbiol 2008;46(1):43–9.

54. del Pozo J, Garcia-Quetglas E, Henaez S, et al. *Granulicatella adiacens* breast implant-associated infection. Diagn Microbiol Infect Dis 2008;61:58–60.

55. Tian H, Tan S, Tay K. Delayed fungal infection following augmentation mammoplasty in an immunocompetent host. Singapore Med J 2007;48(3):256–8.

56. Wright P, Raine C, Ragbir M, et al. The semi-permeability of silicone: a saline-filled breast implant with intraluminal and pericapsular *Aspergillus flavus*. J Plast Reconstr Aesthet Surg 2006;59:1118–21.

57. Niazi Z, Niazi M, Salzberg C, et al. *Candida albicans* infection of bilateral polyurethane-coated silicone gel breast implants. Ann Plast Surg 1996;37:91–3.

58. Rieger U, Pierer G, Luscher M, et al. Sonification of removed breast implants for improved detection of subclinical infection. Aesthetic Plast Surg 2009;33(3):404–8.

59. del Pozo J, Tran N, Petty P, et al. Pilot study of association of bacteria on breast implants with capsular contracture. J Clin Microbiol 2009;47(5):1333–7.

60. Tambuto H, Vickery K, Deva A. Subclinical (biofilm) infection causes capsular contracture in a porcine model following augmentation mammaplasty. Plast Reconstr Surg 2010;126(3):835–42.

61. Carlesimo B, Cigna E, Fino P, et al. Antibiotic therapy of transaxillary augmentation mammoplasty. In Vivo 2009;23(2):357–62.

62. Administration FaD. Anaplastic large cell lymphoma (ACLC) in women with breast implants: Preliminary FDA finding and analysis. 2011. Available at: http://www.fda.gov/MedicalDevices/ProductsandMedicalProcedures/ImplantsandProsthetics/BreastImplants/ucm239996.htm#recommendations. Accessed June 10, 2011.

63. Griffith D, Aksamit T, Brown-Elliot B, et al. An official ATS/IDSA statement: diagnosis, treatment, and prevention of nontuberculous mycobacterial diseases. Am J Respir Crit Care Med 2007;175:367–416.

64. Halvorson E, Disa J, Mehrara B, et al. Outcome following removal of infected tissue expanders in breast reconstruction: a 10-year experience. Ann Plast Surg 2007;59:131–6.

65. Spear S, Howard M, Boehmler J, et al. The infected or exposed breast implant: management and treatment strategies. Plast Reconstr Surg 2004;113:1634–44.

66. Laveaux C, Pauchot J, Loury J, et al. Acute periprosthetic infection after aesthetic breast augmentation. Report of three cases of implant "salvage". Proposal of a standardized protocol of care. Ann Chir Plast Esthet 2009;54(4):358–64.

67. Kendrick A, Chase C. Salvage of an infected breast tissue expander with an implant sizer and negative pressure wound management. Plast Reconstr Surg 2008;121(3):138e–9e.

68. Spear S, Seruya M. Management of the infected or exposed breast prosthesis: a single surgeon's 15-year experience with 69 patients. Plast Reconstr Surg 2010;125:1074–84.

69. Margakis L, Perl T. Basics of surgical site infection surveillance and prevention. In: Lautenbach E, Woeltje K, Malani P, editors. The Society for Healthcare Epidemiology of America practical healthcare epidemiology. 3rd edition. Chicago: University of Chicago Press; 2010. p. 173–85.

70. Mangram A, Horan T, Pearson M, et al. Guideline for prevention of surgical site infection, 1999. Infect Control Hosp Epidemiol 1999;20(4):247–78.

71. Tejirian T, DiFronzo L, Haigh P. Antibiotic prophylaxis for preventing wound infection after breast surgery: a systematic review and metaanalysis. J Am Coll Surg 2006;203(5):729–34.
72. Cunningham M, Bunn F, Handscomb K. Prophylactic antibiotics to prevent surgical site infection after breast cancer surgery. Cochrane Database Syst Rev 2006;2:CD005360.
73. Clegg H, Bertagnoli P, Hightower A, et al. Mammaplasty-associated mycobacterial infection: a survey of plastic surgeons. Plast Reconstr Surg 1983;72(2):165–9.
74. Gordon S. Antibiotic prophylaxis against postoperative wound infections. Cleve Clin J Med 2006;73(Suppl 1):S42–5.
75. Antimicrobial prophylaxis for surgery. Treat Guidel Med Lett 2009;7(82):47–52.
76. Bratzler D, Houck P. Antimicrobial prophylaxis for surgery: an advisory statement from the National Surgical Infection Prevention Project. Am J Surg 2005;189: 395–404.
77. Phillips B, Wang E, Mirrer J, et al. Current practice among plastic surgeons of antibiotic prophylaxis and closed-suction drains in breast reconstruction. Ann Plast Surg 2011;66(5):460–5.
78. Throckmorton A, Hoskin T, Boostrom S, et al. Complications associated with postoperative antibiotic prophylaxis after breast surgery. Am J Surg 2009;198(4): 553–6.
79. Khan U. Breast augmentation, antibiotic prophylaxis, and infection: comparative analysis of 1,628 primary augmentation mammoplasties assessing the role and efficacy of antibiotics prophylaxis duration. Aesthetic Plast Surg 2010;34:42–7.
80. Chundamala M, Wright J. The efficacy and risks of using povidone-iodine irrigation to prevent surgical site infection: an evidence-based review. Can J Surg 2007;50(6):473–81.
81. Administration FaD. 2000. Available at: http://www.fda.gov/MedicalDevices/ProductsandIProcedures/ImplantsandProsthetics/BreastImplants/ucm063860.htm. Accessed May 19, 2011.
82. McHugh S, Collins C, Corrigan M, et al. The role of topical antibiotics used as prophylaxis in surgical site infection prevention. J Antimicrob Chemother 2011; 66:693–701.
83. Adams W, Rios J, Smith S. Enhancing patient outcomes in aesthetic and reconstructive breast surgery using triple antibiotic breast irrigation: six-year prospective clinical study. Plast Reconstr Surg 2006;117:30–6.
84. Burkhardt B, Dempsey P, Schnur P, et al. Capsular contracture: a prospective study of the effect of local antibacterial agents. Plast Reconstr Surg 1986; 77(6):919–30.
85. Darouiche R, Netscher D, Mansouri M, et al. Activity of antimicrobial-impregnated silicone tissue expanders. Ann Plast Surg 2002;49(6):567–71.

Infectious Complications of Dialysis Access Devices

Natasha Bagdasarian, MD, MPH[a,b,]*, Michael Heung, MD, MS[c],
Preeti N. Malani, MD, MSJ[d]

KEYWORDS

• Dialysis • Device infection • Renal disease

During the past 2 decades, the incidence of end-stage renal disease (ESRD) in the United States has more than doubled, with more than 380,000 patients currently receiving maintenance dialysis.[1] During this same time period, significant advances have been made in dialysis care and overall survival.[1] However, dialysis access can be problematic, including vascular access for hemodialysis (HD) and peritoneal access for peritoneal dialysis (PD). Dialysis access remains the Achilles heel of ESRD management, and represents a major source of morbidity for these patients while contributing significantly to health care costs.

Infections are a significant, potentially modifiable, contributor to access-related difficulties. In general, infections represent the second leading cause of death in ESRD patients, behind only cardiovascular disease, and are a leading cause of hospitalization.[1–4] Between 2007 and 2008, HD patients experienced a rate of 0.47 infection-related hospitalizations per patient-year, reflecting an almost 50% increase since 1993.[1] Similarly, albeit to a lesser degree, the rate of infection-related hospitalization has increased by 7.5% in PD patients.[1] The rate of hospitalization specifically

There was no outside support for this work.

The authors have nothing to disclose.

[a] Division of General Medicine, University of Michigan and Veterans Affairs Ann Arbor Healthcare System, 2215 Fuller Road, Ann Arbor, MI 48105, USA

[b] Division of Infectious Diseases, University of Michigan and Veterans Affairs Ann Arbor Healthcare System, 2215 Fuller Road, Ann Arbor, MI 48105, USA

[c] Division of Nephrology, University of Michigan, 1500 East Medical Center Drive, Ann Arbor, MI 48109, USA

[d] Department of Internal Medicine, Divisions of Infectious Diseases and Geriatric Medicine, University of Michigan and Ann Arbor Veterans Affairs Ann Arbor Healthcare System, Geriatric Research Education and Clinical Center, 2215 Fuller Road, 111-I, 8th Floor, Ann Arbor, MI 48105, USA

* Corresponding author. VA Healthcare System, 2215 Fuller Road, Ann Arbor, MI 48105.

E-mail address: nghazi@umich.edu

Infect Dis Clin N Am 26 (2012) 127–141

doi:10.1016/j.idc.2011.09.005

0891-5520/12/$ – see front matter Published by Elsevier Inc.

for vascular access–related infections has improved but remains at 0.11 per patient-year.[1] There clearly remains much room for improvement.

In this review the authors consider the important infectious complications associated with dialysis access. The discussion includes the epidemiology, microbiology, management, and outcomes related to dialysis-access infections.

HEMODIALYSIS ACCESS

More than 90% of prevalent maintenance dialysis patients in the United States (more than 350,000 patients) undergo HD therapy, with the vast majority receiving in-center dialysis thrice weekly.[1] Infectious complications contribute significantly to the morbidity and mortality of these patients.

Patients with chronic kidney disease (CKD) are at higher risk of bacteremia than those without CKD, and patients requiring hemodialysis are at even higher risk of systemic infection.[5] Uremia-associated phagocyte dysfunction, iron overload, and comorbidities including diabetes mellitus, can affect host immunity. Additional risk factors for bacteremia in HD patients include a previous history of bacteremia, receipt of immunosuppressive therapy, anemia, and hepatitis C infection.[6,7] However, one of the most significant risk factors for infection is the type of HD access used, which is a potentially modifiable risk factor.

Table 1 provides an overview of the different vascular access options available for HD patients. The risk of access-related infection is highest for nontunneled catheters, followed by tunneled catheters and then arteriovenous grafts (AVGs), while arteriovenous fistulas (AVFs) have the lowest overall risk of infection.[6,8–12] A large, multicenter, prospective study found the rate of bloodstream infection with AVFs was 0.2 per 1000 dialysis procedures, and the relative risk of infection was 2.5 with AVGs, 15.5 with tunneled catheters, and 22.5 with nontunneled catheters.[9]

The primary preferred access is an AVF, due to its low risk of infection and high long-term patency rates. However, AVFs typically require 2 to 3 months to mature after surgical creation, and primary failure rates are high. As a result, less than 20% of new ESRD patients initiate maintenance dialysis with AVFs.[1] To address this, in 2004 the Centers for Medicare and Medicaid Services introduced the national "Fistula First Initiative," and during the past several years the use of AVFs in the overall HD population has improved from 32.2% in 2003 to 55.8% in 2010.[13]

After an AVF, the next best option is generally considered to be an AVG, in which an artery is connected to a vein using exogenous material, most commonly polytetrafluoroethylene. The advantages of an AVG over an AVF include less maturation time (typically 3–4 weeks after placement or even immediate use with newer graft materials) and lower primary failure rates. However, an AVG involves implantation of a foreign body and therefore has a higher infection risk. There is also a higher risk of access-related thrombosis and lower average access life span compared with an AVF. This access type is generally considered when an AVF is not feasible because of poor endogenous veins. In some cases, graft material is also placed as a patch to salvage a nonmaturing AVF.

Hemodialysis catheters are associated with the highest incidence of complications, particularly infection, and are therefore considered the least favorable option for HD access.[1,14,15] More than 80% of incident ESRD patients in the United States start hemodialysis with catheter access, in stark contrast to rates in other industrialized nations (23% in Germany and 29% in Japan).[16]

During the first 6 months of dialysis patients with catheters have higher hospitalization rates, especially for infection-related complications, and the relative risk of sepsis

Table 1
Vascular access options for hemodialysis patients

Access Type	Description	Primary Indication	Pros	Cons	Relative Infectious Risk[a]
Arteriovenous fistula (AVF)	Surgical connection created between native artery and vein	Preferred access of choice for ESRD patients undergoing HD	Highest long-term patency rate Associated with lowest mortality compared with other access options	Long maturation period (typically 2–3 mo) High primary failure rate	1
Arteriovenous graft (AVG)	Exogenous tube placed subcutaneously to connect artery and vein	Second choice access for ESRD patients undergoing HD	Faster maturation (3–4 wk after placement) Higher early patency rates than AVF	Higher infectious risk than AVF Lower long-term patency rate than AVF	2
Tunneled dialysis catheter	Central venous catheter with subcutaneous tract between vascular insertion and skin exit	For patients who do not have a mature AVF or AVG at time of HD initiation	Immediate use	High infection risk Flow problems due to clotting, fibrin sheaths, malposition	3
Acute (nontunneled) dialysis catheter	Central venous catheter	Reserved for in-hospital acute HD; temporary access only	Easy placement without need for fluoroscopy Immediate use	Highest risk for infection	4

Abbreviations: ESRD, end-stage renal disease; HD, hemodialysis.
[a] Relative infectious risk: 1 = lowest, 4 = highest.

is higher.[6,15] Mortality is also higher, and this difference is especially pronounced in older adults.[17] While the issue of catheter-related infection affects all patients with central venous catheters (CVCs), it is of particular importance to patients receiving HD. This aspect was highlighted in a recent report by the Centers for Disease Control and Prevention (CDC) showing that, whereas catheter-related bloodstream infections (CRBSI) in intensive care units have decreased over the past decade, CRBSI rates in dialysis units remain high.[16]

There are two main types of HD catheter: tunneled and nontunneled. Nontunneled catheters are the easiest access to place for immediate dialysis needs and therefore represent the most common access type used in patients with acute kidney injury requiring hemodialysis therapy. These catheters also have the highest infection rate, due to the direct connection between the bloodstream and skin surface. Tunneled catheters are associated with a lower risk of infection because of the creation of a subcutaneous tract (typically at least 10 cm) between the vascular insertion site and the cutaneous exit site. If temporary dialysis access is needed but the catheter is expected to stay in place for more than 2 to 3 weeks, a tunneled catheter is preferable to a nontunneled catheter.[8,18]

The site of an HD catheter may also play a role in the relative risk of infection. Femoral catheters are generally believed to be associated with a higher risk of infection, followed by internal jugular and then subclavian catheters.[8,19] However, one large, randomized, multicenter study found that jugular catheters did not reduce the risk of infection compared with femoral catheters, except among adults with a high body mass index (>28.4 kg/m^2).[20]

Clinical Manifestations and Diagnosis

Exit-site infections (ESIs) are characterized by erythema, tenderness, induration, or purulence at the CVC exit site, while tunnel infections (TIs) are characterized by signs of infection extending greater than 2 cm from the exit site.[18] ESIs and TIs may occur concurrently with CRBSIs, especially with *Staphylococcus aureus* infections.[21]

According to the Infectious Disease Society of America (IDSA) guidelines, diagnosis of CRBSI requires either growth of the same organism from a percutaneous blood culture and from a catheter tip culture, or that two blood samples (one sample from a catheter and the other from a peripheral vein) meet quantitative or differential time to positivity (DTP) criteria.[22] Quantitative blood cultures are defined by blood drawn through the catheter demonstrating a bacterial colony count 3 times greater than blood drawn peripherally, while DTP requires that bacterial growth from catheter-drawn blood occurs 2 hours before blood drawn from a peripheral vein.[22] For both of these criteria it is important to ensure that the same volume of blood has been inserted into each culture bottle. Blood cultures should be drawn before initiating treatment because receipt of antimicrobials can decrease the sensitivity.

These testing paradigms may be difficult to adhere to for practical reasons. HD catheters are often not immediately removed when infection is suspected, patients may have limited peripheral vascular access for blood draws, and quantitative or DTP criteria can be problematic for a variety of other logistic reasons. Therefore, CRBSI in hemodialysis patients is often presumed without these strict standards being met. When a symptomatic patient with an indwelling HD catheter has positive catheter-drawn and/or peripheral blood culture, with no other identifiable source of infection, CRBSI may be presumed.[22] If blood cannot be drawn peripherally, samples may be drawn through multiple catheter lumens. Positive blood cultures and evidence of exit-site or tunnel infection can also indicate CRBSI, and drainage at the exit site should be cultured if present.

AVG or AVF infections can present with erythema, pain, and warmth at the access site, though this is not always the case. Imaging may be helpful for patients with bacteremia and arteriovenous access. Some experts advocate the use of indium scans to diagnose occult arteriovenous access infections when there is high clinical suspicion,[23] although the sensitivity and specificity of this approach is not well established.

It may be difficult to tell whether a single positive blood culture represents true infection rather than contamination. In general, certain virulent organisms (ie, *S aureus*) should never be treated as contaminants, whereas less virulent organisms (ie, coagulase-negative *Staphylococcus*) may be considered contaminants if the patient is asymptomatic and repeat blood cultures remain negative.

Epidemiology and Microbiology

Although gram-negative and fungal CRBSIs do occur, gram-positive cocci make up the vast majority of HD-related infections. Most cases are attributable to *S aureus* and coagulase-negative *Staphylococcus* (CoNS), but enterococcal infections also occur.[6,9,24] The microbiology appears to vary by access type. Nontunneled catheter–associated CRBSIs are caused most often by CoNS, followed by *S aureus*, *Candida* species, enteric gram-negative bacilli (GNB), *Pseudomonas*, and enterococci.[25] Tunneled catheter CRBSI are caused most often by CoNS, followed by enteric GNB, *S aureus*, *Pseudomonas*, enterococci, and *Candida*.[25] Whereas CoNS is responsible for most CVC infections, *S aureus* is more common with AVF and AVG infections.[11] *S aureus* is more often associated with treatment failure and infectious complications of CRBSI.[26]

Infections with antimicrobial resistant organisms are a growing concern among dialysis patients. In 2005, the incidence of invasive methicillin-resistant *S aureus* (MRSA) infection among dialysis patients was 45.2 cases per 1000 population, compared with rates in the general population that have ranged from 0.2 to 0.4 infections per 1000 population.[27] Infections with vancomycin-resistant enterococci (VRE) also remain a challenge. VRE bloodstream infections are associated with hemodialysis, and among dialysis-dependent patients risk factors for VRE colonization include previous antimicrobial use, specifically β-lactams, and extended durations of hospitalization.[28,29] Furthermore, vancomycin-intermediate *S aureus* (VISA) infections have been reported among hemodialysis patients; often after extended exposure to vancomycin for MRSA infections.[30,31] Vancomycin-resistant *S aureus* (VRSA) strains are an emerging issue in parts of the United States, and may become a bigger concern among HD patients in the future.[32] Azole-resistant *Candida* species are associated with many HD-related infections, and non-*albicans Candida* species (particularly *C glabrata* and *C krusei*), are responsible for more episodes of fungemia among HD patients than in non-HD patients (31% vs 17%).[33]

Hematogenous complications of CRBSI include endocarditis, osteomyelitis, epidural abscess, and septic arthritis.[26,34,35] Hemodialysis dependence is a risk factor for complications of CRBSI, as is the presence of a long-term intravascular catheter and attempt at catheter salvage.[26,36] MRSA has a particular propensity to cause hematogenous complications.[21,26,36] In patients with prolonged bacteremia or fungemia, particularly after hemodialysis catheter removal, other foci of infection should be suspected.

Treatment

The general approach toward a patient with fever and an indwelling HD catheter is to first obtain blood cultures, then consider initiating antimicrobial therapy and removing the catheter, depending on the clinical scenario. This approach is often complicated by limited vascular access sites and the ongoing need for HD.

The approach to empiric antimicrobial choice among dialysis patients is beyond the scope of this article; however, a few key points are summarized here. Vancomycin is the preferred empiric therapy for CRBSI in heath care settings with an elevated prevalence of MRSA, whereas daptomycin is preferred in settings where vancomycin minimum inhibitory concentration values greater than 2 mg/mL are common. Empiric coverage for GNB therapy should be used in critically ill patients and patients with femoral lines, and coverage for multidrug-resistant (MDR) GNB should be considered in immunocompromised patients, critically ill or septic patents, or patients with a history of MDR GNB infections or colonization. Coverage for *Candida* species should be considered in critically ill patients with a femoral line and in immunosuppressed patients, with use of total parenteral nutrition (TPN) or prolonged use of broad-spectrum antibiotics, or colonization with *Candida* species at multiple sites.[22]

Optimal dosing of antimicrobials can be problematic in dialysis patients. For example, vancomycin dosing can be affected by the type of dialysis filter used, duration of and intervals between dialysis sessions, body weight, and residual renal function; and while low levels can be associated with treatment failures and the emergence of drug resistance, high levels have been associated with increased risk of nephrotoxicity and ototoxicity.[37] Duration of antimicrobial therapy depends on the clinical scenario and presence of other foci of infection.

In most situations, the ideal approach to catheter-related infections includes antimicrobial therapy along with prompt removal of the catheter followed by a line-free interval before catheter replacement in a different site. Unfortunately, such an approach is complicated by a variety of issues unique to HD patients. First, the possibility of a line-free interval is limited by dialysis needs. In addition, HD catheters are often seen as a patient's life-line, and the risk of losing vascular access altogether can result in hesitance toward early catheter removal. Some HD patients have extremely limited access options, and failure to establish new access represents a terminal complication. As such, a frequent approach is to try to salvage the dialysis access.

Although it is generally accepted that catheter salvage is not advisable for *S aureus* or *Candida* infections, salvage may be successful in certain situations. In uncomplicated CRBSI involving organisms that are relatively easy to eradicate, such as CoNS, treatment may be attempted without catheter removal. A recent retrospective study concluded that catheter salvage may be possible in CRBSI caused by CoNS, even with concurrent ESI.[21] However, IDSA guidelines recommend removing long-term catheters in the setting of sepsis, tunnel infection, or hematogenous spread of infection.[22] Other indications for removal of tunneled HD catheters include failure to clear blood cultures after 72 hours of therapy, or for infections due to *S aureus, Pseudomonas aeruginosa,* fungi, mycobacteria, or other bacteria difficult to eradicate (*Bacillus, Micrococcus,* or Propionibacteria).[22] Most studies have shown that catheter salvage has a 25% to 33% chance of success.[35,38] An observational study of 226 patients with tunneled-catheter infections found that HD catheter salvage resulted in an overall fourfold higher risk of treatment failure, and an eightfold higher risk of treatment failure in patients with *S aureus* infections.[26]

Another prospective study evaluated attempted salvage of infected tunneled dialysis catheters in 154 patients with clinical response to antimicrobials within 48 hours.[39] Two-thirds of cases demonstrated no recurrence or complications during the 6-month follow-up period, although salvage was only attempted in 74% of cases and treatment durations were long (6 weeks). No differences in outcome were observed based on the organism isolated; however, no cases of candidemia were included in the catheter-salvage group. Infection recurrence tended to occur in the second month following attempted catheter salvage, and success decreased with each subsequent attempt at catheter salvage. Clinicians must be aware that although catheter salvage is appropriate in some cases, such an approach frequently results in worse outcomes.

In certain situations, catheter exchange over a guide wire may be the only feasible way to replace a dialysis catheter without risk of losing vascular access entirely. Although CDC guidelines do not recommend guide-wire exchanges for catheter-related infections,[18] some data suggest that guide-wire exchange may reduce secondary vertebral or paraspinal infections compared with no exchange,[40] and another study suggested that outcomes do not differ when comparing tunneled-catheter exchange over a guide wire versus catheter removal and delayed replacement.[26] A retrospective study of 40 HD patients with candidemia compared catheter exchange over a guide wire to catheter removal with delayed replacement and found similar outcomes between the two groups, concluding that guide-wire exchange may be an effective option for HD patients with candidemia.[41] These data should be interpreted with caution, as fungal CRBSIs are more likely to result in relapse of infection, even after tunneled-catheter removal and reinsertion.[42]

Though rare, AVG infections can occur, and infection accounts for more than one-third of AVG losses or failures.[43] As with HD catheters, the decision to remove an infected AVG is often not pursued aggressively, in favor of a more conservative approach comprising antimicrobial therapy and attempted salvage. In general, the decision to pursue AVG removal must consider the urgency of the clinical picture, and balance the competing risks of a potentially worse infectious complication (such as sepsis or hematogenous complications) versus the loss of HD access and resultant commitment to catheter access for a minimum of 2 months. Graft removal is indicated with extensive infection if infection occurs before the graft has become embedded, or in septic patients.[11] Partial AVG excision with access salvage has been found to be a reasonable option in patients with localized abscess or generally more limited infection.[43,44]

Prevention

As already mentioned, the most significant approach to HD access infection prevention has been the major push to promote AVF use and limit HD catheter use. Despite these efforts, a significant proportion of prevalent HD patients remain catheter dependent. In these patients, several preventive strategies have been used.

The use of topical antimicrobials at the CVC exit site has been suggested as a strategy to decrease infectious risk among HD patients. A 2010 Cochrane review concluded that use of topical mupirocin ointment reduced the risk of CRBSI in patients on HD, while there was insufficient evidence to support the role of topical honey, povidone-iodine ointment, polysporin ointment, or various types of dressing to reduce the risk of catheter-related infections.[45] However, a recent study found that the use of topical polyantibiotic ointment was associated a with decrease in CVC-related infections,[46] and the 2011 CDC guidelines for prevention of CRBSI recommend the routine use of povidone-iodine antiseptic ointment or polyantibiotic ointment at the HD catheter exit site at the end of each dialysis session,[18] although its use may be limited by instances of contact dermatitis.

There is much literature regarding the use of antimicrobial-impregnated catheters in the intensive care unit, and CDC guidelines recommend the use of these antimicrobial-coated CVCs in populations with high rates of catheter-related infections.[18] A prospective study using minocycline/rifampin-coated HD catheters showed decreased rates of infection in patients with acute kidney injury[47]; however, this practice has not been widely studied in the chronic dialysis population. Indeed, this approach may be impractical because of the higher costs associated with these catheters. The data on silver-coated dialysis catheters have been mixed. A prospective, randomized study looking at silver-coated tunneled dialysis catheters did not find a reduction in infection or colonization,[48] but a second prospective study found decreased bacterial colonization on the silver-coated catheter.[49]

Antimicrobial locks are another strategy to reduce the risk of recurrent infection among catheter-dependent patients, including those receiving HD. The most recent guidelines recommend considering using lock therapy among patients who develop recurrent infections despite optimal adherence to aseptic technique.[18] The technique involves filling the catheter lumen with a lock solution and allowing it to dwell when the catheter is not in use. Lock solutions include antibiotics (most often vancomycin or an aminoglycoside) as well as other agents (ie, ethanol and recombinant tissue plasminogen activator). Gentamicin/heparin and taurolidine/citrate catheter locks have been shown to reduce rates of CRBSI when compared with heparin alone; however, gentamicin can be associated with ototoxicity, and taurolidine is not available in the United States.[50] Recently, a novel lock solution containing sodium citrate, methylene blue, methylparaben, and propylparaben (C-MB-P) has shown promise among HD patients.[51] A multicenter, randomized trial demonstrated that catheters locked with C-MB-P were significantly less likely to be associated with CRBSI. The cost-effectiveness of antimicrobial locks has not been fully evaluated, and this approach carries the risk of increasing antimicrobial resistance. Further studies are needed to confirm these results and to determine whether this approach should be applied on a larger scale.

PERITONEAL DIALYSIS ACCESS

Among incident ESRD patients, only 6% choose peritoneal dialysis as their initial modality.[1] In contrast to HD, the only access option for PD is a tunneled PD catheter. Patients undergoing PD are at risk of PD catheter–related peritonitis, ESIs, or TIs. During the past 2 decades the rate of PD-associated infections has improved dramatically, but peritonitis remains the most common cause of PD failure, leading to transfer to HD.[1]

While sharing the same underlying risk characteristics as HD patients, PD patients face different challenges specific to their chosen dialysis modality. Although PD patients do not have indwelling vascular access, the near constant dwell of a dextrose-rich solution in the peritoneal space provides a high-risk environment for infection. PD catheters are accessed multiple times daily, in contrast to the thrice weekly use of HD catheters. Lastly, PD patients must rely on themselves (or their caregivers) to maintain sterile technique and avoid contamination, whereas HD patients are managed by trained technicians and nurses. Nevertheless, with appropriate training and motivation, PD can be performed with great success and relatively few infectious complications.

Older patients, females, and smokers appear to be at higher risk of PD-associated peritonitis.[52] The choice of PD fluid may affect the risk of infection, and solutions with low concentrations of glucose degradation products may be associated with decreased infection rates, although data are inconclusive.[53] The location of abdominally placed peritoneal catheters may contribute to infectious risk, and presternal placement of peritoneal catheters may have a lower risk of infection.[54] Certain dialysate bag systems (Y-set bag systems versus double-bag systems) may also be associated with higher risk of peritonitis.[55] Recently published data suggest that automated PD, defined as use of a machine to do exchanges, typically overnight, is associated with a lower risk of infection than is continuous ambulatory PD, although it is unclear whether this is related to the connection system used or the number of times the catheter is accessed.[56]

Clinical Manifestations and Diagnosis

PD-associated ESIs are characterized by purulent drainage and erythema surrounding the catheter. PD-associated TIs are characterized by erythema, edema, or tenderness over the catheter tunnel, and usually occur in conjunction with an ESI, especially with *S aureus* and *P aeruginosa*. Cultures from the PD catheter exit site should only be obtained when there is clinical suspicion of infection, as a positive culture alone may simply represent colonization.

Patients on PD with cloudy effluent and/or abdominal pain should be evaluated for peritonitis. According to the International Society for Peritoneal Dialysis guidelines, PD-associated peritonitis (PDP) is defined as any 2 of the following: (1) signs and symptoms consistent with PDP; (2) white blood cell count greater than 100/mL in PD effluent and greater than 50% neutrophils after a dwell time of at least 2 hours; and (3) a positive culture of an organism from the PD effluent.[57] While Gram stain and culture should be performed to help guide therapy, cultures are often negative.[57,58] Leukocyte esterase strips have shown promise for the detection of PDP, with sensitivity approaching 100% and specificity greater than 95%.[59]

Epidemiology and Microbiology

PD-associated infections are most commonly caused by CoNS, which accounts for approximately 30% of cases, followed by nonpseudomonal Gram negatives and *S aureus*; while 10% to 30% of cases are culture negative.[58,60,61] Patients with culture-negative PDP are more likely to have had recent antimicrobial exposure.[62] Fungal peritonitis occurs in fewer than 5% of cases of PDP; it is typically caused by *Candida* species and is commonly preceded by antimicrobial use.[63,64] Poor outcome and PDP-related morbidity is typically associated with gram-negative stain, and fungal peritonitis.[57,65] Pseudomonal peritonitis, in particular, is associated with higher frequency of ESI and TI, higher hospitalization rates, increased catheter loss, and lower rates of cure.[66]

Resistant gram-positive organisms, including VISA, have been associated with PDP-related peritonitis, notably in patients who have had long courses of antimicrobials. In fact, one of the first documented cases of VISA infection was in a PD-dependent patient who had previously been treated with 18 weeks of vancomycin for recurrent MRSA PDP.[67]

Treatment and Prevention

After obtaining fluid for cell count, Gram stain, and culture, antimicrobials should be started as soon as possible for suspected cases of PDP. Empiric therapy for PD catheter–associated ESIs or TIs should include coverage for *S aureus*, and local resistance patterns may indicate a need for MRSA coverage. Gram-negative organisms, including *Pseudomonas*, may also cause PDP, and therapy should be tailored depending on culture results. Intraperitoneal antimicrobials are typically preferred for PDP and hold the major advantage of not requiring additional intravenous access as compared with parenteral administration. Vancomycin, cephalosporins, and aminoglycosides all have demonstrated stability and bioactivity in PD solution. However, certain agents cannot be mixed in the same bag, and care should be taken to ensure compatibility of intraperitoneal antimicrobials infused together. In addition, to ensure appropriate absorption of the drug, intraperitoneal dwell time should be at least 6 hours. Specifics on antimicrobial choice and dosing are beyond the scope of this review but are discussed elsewhere.[68–70]

Catheters can usually be salvaged for culture-negative or CoNS PDP, but catheter removal is typically required in cases of refractory or relapsing peritonitis; *Pseudomonas*, *S aureus*, or fungal peritonitis; and peritonitis with TI or ESI.[57,62,71] When catheter removal is indicated, simultaneous insertion of a new PD catheter is often successful, although some data suggest that this approach is less successful during active infection, and for *Pseudomonas* or fungal peritonitis.[72–74]

Complicated PDP is associated with concurrent ESI, elevated effluent white cell count after 3 to 5 days of treatment, and low serum protein level.[60,75] Ultrasonography may be used to predict treatment failure, and a lucency of greater than 1 mm around the external cuff, following antimicrobial treatment, has been associated with poor clinical outcome.[76] Other factors associated with treatment failure include diabetes mellitus and Pseudomonal, fungal, or mycobacterial peritonitis.[65,66,77]

Isolation of multiple enteric organisms may indicate underlying intra-abdominal pathology including diverticulitis, cholecystitis, ischemic bowel, and appendicitis, and are associated with an increased risk of death.[57] Prompt surgical evaluation should be considered in these situations.

Topical mupirocin application has been used to prevent PDP and ESI, with some success.[78] Although data from animal models have been promising, data on the use of antimicrobial-coated PD catheters in humans are mixed. A randomized, prospective study evaluating silver-coated PD catheters did not show any reduction in PDP or ESI rates.[79] There have been some data to support use of prophylactic fluconazole in patients with bacterial PDP to prevent subsequent fungal peritonitis, although this practice is not common.[63,80]

SUMMARY

Despite overall progress, access-associated infections remain a major source of morbidity and mortality among dialysis patients. In HD patients the risk may be modifiable with appropriate access planning, but in PD patients the risk factors for infection are less well understood. In both groups, gram-positive cocci account for the majority of infections, although gram-negative infections are not uncommon and resistant organisms represent a growing concern. In addition, practitioners should be aware of the unique issues surrounding dialysis access, namely that access represents a life-line for ESRD patients. A decision for early access removal must recognize the potential risks of losing dialysis access; conversely, a decision to treat through and salvage an access must be carefully weighed against the risk of greater infectious complications. Such therapeutic decision making must be individualized to each patient's specific situation.

ACKNOWLEDGMENTS

The authors thank Jonathan H. Segal, MD for his thoughtful review of this work.

REFERENCES

1. U S Renal Data System, USRDS 2010 annual data report: atlas of chronic kidney disease and end-stage renal disease in the united states. Bethesda (MD): National

Institutes of Health, National Institute of Diabetes and Digestive and Kidney Diseases; 2010.

2. Patel PR, Kallen AJ, Arduino MJ. Epidemiology, surveillance, and prevention of bloodstream infections in hemodialysis patients. Am J Kidney Dis 2010;56:566–77.

3. Gallieni M, Martini A, Mezzina N. Dialysis access: an increasingly important clinical issue. Int J Artif Organs 2009;32:851–6.

4. Fitzgibbons LN, Puls DL, Mackay K, et al. Management of gram-positive coccal bacteremia and hemodialysis. Am J Kidney Dis 2011;57:624–40.

5. James MT, Laupland KB, Tonelli M, et al. Risk of bloodstream infection in patients with chronic kidney disease not treated with dialysis. Arch Intern Med 2008;168: 2333–9.

6. Hoen B, Paul-Dauphin A, Hestin D, et al. EPIBACDIAL: a multicenter prospective study of risk factors for bacteremia in chronic hemodialysis patients. J Am Soc Nephrol 1998;9:869–76.

7. Reddy S, Sullivan R, Zaiden R, et al. Hepatitis C infection and the risk of bacteremia in hemodialysis patients with tunneled vascular access catheters. South Med J 2009;102:374–7.

8. Weijmer MC, Vervloet MG, ter Wee PM. Compared to tunnelled cuffed haemodialysis catheters, temporary untunnelled catheters are associated with more complications already within 2 weeks of use. Nephrol Dial Transplant 2004;19:670–7.

9. Taylor G, Gravel D, Johnston L, et al. Prospective surveillance for primary bloodstream infections occurring in Canadian hemodialysis units. Infect Control Hosp Epidemiol 2002;23:716–20.

10. Schild AF, Perez E, Gillaspie E, et al. Arteriovenous fistulae vs. arteriovenous grafts: a retrospective review of 1,700 consecutive vascular access cases. J Vasc Access 2008;9:231–5.

11. Akoh JA. Vascular access infections: epidemiology, diagnosis, and management. Curr Infect Dis Rep 2011;13(4):324–32.

12. Yu Q, Yu H, Chen S, et al. Distribution and complications of native arteriovenous fistulas in maintenance hemodialysis patients: a single-center study. J Nephrol 2011;24(5):597–603.

13. Wish JB. Vascular access for dialysis in the United States: progress, hurdles, controversies, and the future. Semin Dial 2010;23:614–8.

14. Betjes MG. Prevention of catheter-related bloodstream infection in patients on hemodialysis. Nat Rev Nephrol 2011;7:257–65.

15. Ng LJ, Chen F, Pisoni RL, et al. Hospitalization risks related to vascular access type among incident US hemodialysis patients. Nephrol Dial Transplant 2011. [Epub ahead of print].

16. Centers for Disease Control and Prevention (CDC). Vital signs: central line-associated blood stream infections—United States, 2001, 2008, and 2009. MMWR Morb Mortal Wkly Rep 2011;60:243–8.

17. Ocak G, Halbesma N, le Cessie S, et al. Haemodialysis catheters increase mortality as compared to arteriovenous accesses especially in elderly patients. Nephrol Dial Transplant 2011;26(8):2611–7.

18. O'Grady NP, Alexander M, Burns LA, et al. Guidelines for the prevention of intravascular catheter-related infections. Clin Infect Dis 2011;52:e162–93.

19. Kairaitis LK, Gottlieb T. Outcome and complications of temporary haemodialysis catheters. Nephrol Dial Transplant 1999;14:1710–4.

20. Parienti JJ, Thirion M, Mégarbane B, et al. Femoral vs jugular venous catheterization and risk of nosocomial events in adults requiring acute renal replacement therapy: a randomized controlled trial. JAMA 2008;299:2413–22.

21. Sychev D, Maya ID, Allon M. Clinical management of dialysis catheter-related bacteremia with concurrent exit-site infection. Semin Dial 2011;24:239–41.
22. Mermel LA, Allon M, Bouza E, et al. Clinical practice guidelines for the diagnosis and management of intravascular catheter-related infection: 2009 update by the Infectious Diseases Society of America. Clin Infect Dis 2009;49:1–45.
23. Nassar GM, Ayus JC. Infectious complications of the hemodialysis access. Kidney Int 2001;60:1–13.
24. Saeed Abdulrahman I, Al-Mueilo SH, Bokhary HA, et al. prospective study of hemodialysis access-related bacterial infections. J Infect Chemother 2002;8:242–6.
25. Safdar N, Maki DG. The epidemiology of catheter-related infection in the critically ill. In: O'Grady NP, Pittet D, editors. Catheter related infections in the critically ill. New York: Kluwer; 2004. p. 1–23.
26. Mokrzycki MH, Zhang M, Cohen H, et al. Tunnelled haemodialysis catheter bacteraemia: risk factors for bacteraemia recurrence, infectious complications and mortality. Nephrol Dial Transplant 2006;21:1024–31.
27. Centers for Disease Control and Prevention (CDC). Invasive methicillin-resistant *Staphylococcus aureus* infections among dialysis patients–United States, 2005. MMWR Morb Mortal Wkly Rep 2007;56:197–9.
28. Montecalvo MA, Shay DK, Patel P, et al. Bloodstream infections with vancomycin-resistant enterococci. Arch Intern Med 1996;156(13):1458–62.
29. Servais A, Mercadal L, Brossier F, et al. Rapid curbing of a vancomycin-resistant *Enterococcus faecium* outbreak in a nephrology department. Clin J Am Soc Nephrol 2009;4:1559–64.
30. Naimi TS, Anderson D, O'Boyle C, et al. Vancomycin-intermediate *Staphylococcus aureus* with phenotypic susceptibility to methicillin in a patient with recurrent bacteremia. Clin Infect Dis 2003;36:1609–12.
31. Rice LB. Antimicrobial resistance in gram-positive bacteria. Am J Med 2006;119: S11–9.
32. Chang S, Sievert DM, Hageman JC, et al. Infection with vancomycin-resistant *Staphylococcus aureus* containing the vanA resistance gene. N Engl J Med 2003;348:1342–7.
33. Pyrgos V, Ratanavanich K, Donegan N, et al. Candida bloodstream infections in hemodialysis recipients. Med Mycol 2009;47:463–7.
34. Kamalakannan D, Pai RM, Johnson LB, et al. Epidemiology and clinical outcomes of infective endocarditis in hemodialysis patients. Ann Thorac Surg 2007;83:2081–6.
35. Marr KA, Sexton DJ, Conlon PJ, et al. Catheter-related bacteremia and outcome of attempted catheter salvage in patients undergoing hemodialysis. Ann Intern Med 1997;127:275–80.
36. Fowler VG Jr, Justice A, Moore C, et al. Risk factors for hematogenous complications of intravascular catheter-associated *Staphylococcus aureus* bacteremia. Clin Infect Dis 2005;40:695–703.
37. Vandecasteele SJ, De Vriese AS. Vancomycin dosing in patients on intermittent hemodialysis. Semin Dial 2011;24:50–5.
38. Saad TF. Bacteremia associated with tunneled, cuffed hemodialysis catheters. Am J Kidney Dis 1999;34:1114–24.
39. Ashby DR, Power A, Singh S, et al. Bacteremia associated with tunneled hemodialysis catheters: outcome after attempted salvage. Clin J Am Soc Nephrol 2009;4:1601–5.
40. Philipneri M, Al-Aly Z, Amin K, et al. Routine replacement of tunneled, cuffed, hemodialysis catheters eliminates paraspinal/vertebral infections in patients with catheter-associated bacteremia. Am J Nephrol 2003;23:202–7.

41. Sychev D, Maya ID, Allon M. Clinical outcomes of dialysis catheter-related candidemia in hemodialysis patients. Clin J Am Soc Nephrol 2009;4:1102–5.
42. Chin BS, Han SH, Lee HS, et al. Risk factors for recurrent catheter-related infections after catheter-related bloodstream infections. Int J Infect Dis 2010;14: e16–21.
43. Schutte WP, Helmer SD, Salazar L, et al. Surgical treatment of infected prosthetic dialysis arteriovenous grafts: total versus partial graft excision. Am J Surg 2007; 193:385–8.
44. Ryan SV, Calligaro KD, Scharff J, et al. Management of infected prosthetic dialysis arteriovenous grafts. J Vasc Surg 2004;39:73–8.
45. McCann M, Moore ZE. Interventions for preventing infectious complications in haemodialysis patients with central venous catheters. Cochrane Database Syst Rev 2010;(1):CD006894.
46. Battistella M, Bhola C, Lok CE. Long-term follow-up of the Hemodialysis Infection Prevention with Polysporin Ointment (HIPPO) Study: a quality improvement report. Am J Kidney Dis 2011;57:432–41.
47. Chatzinikolaou I, Finkel K, Hanna H, et al. Antibiotic-coated hemodialysis catheters for the prevention of vascular catheter-related infections: a prospective, randomized study. Am J Med 2003;115:352–7.
48. Trerotola SO, Johnson MS, Shah H, et al. Tunneled hemodialysis catheters: use of a silver-coated catheter for prevention of infection–a randomized study. Radiology 1998;207:491–6.
49. Bambauer R, Mestres P, Schiel R, et al. Long-term catheters for apheresis and dialysis with surface treatment with infection resistance and low thrombogenicity. Ther Apher Dial 2003;7:225–31.
50. Filiopoulos V, Hadjiyannakos D, Koutis I, et al. Approaches to prolong the use of uncuffed hemodialysis catheters: results of a randomized trial. Am J Nephrol 2011;33:260–8.
51. Maki DG, Ash SR, Winger RK, et al. A novel antimicrobial and antithrombotic lock solution for hemodialysis catheters: a multi-center, controlled, randomized trial. Crit Care Med 2011;39:613–20.
52. Kotsanas D, Polkinghorne KR, Korman TM, et al. Risk factors for peritoneal dialysis-related peritonitis: can we reduce the incidence and improve patient selection? Nephrology (Carlton) 2007;12:239–45.
53. Diaz-Buxo JA, Himmele R. Strategies to universally improve peritonitis rates, including use of dialysis solutions with low glucose degradation products. Adv Perit Dial 2010;26:37–40.
54. Zimmerman DG. Presternal catheter design—an opportunity to capitalize on catheter immobilization. Adv Perit Dial 2010;26:91–5.
55. Daly CD, Campbell MK, MacLeod AM, et al. Do the Y-set and double-bag systems reduce the incidence of CAPD peritonitis? A systematic review of randomized controlled trials. Nephrol Dial Transplant 2001;16:341–7.
56. Piraino B, Sheth H. Peritonitis—does peritoneal dialysis modality make a difference? Blood Purif 2010;29:145–9.
57. Li PK, Szeto CC, Piraino B, et al. Peritoneal dialysis-related infections recommendations: 2010 update. Perit Dial Int 2010;30(4):393–423.
58. Davenport A. Peritonitis remains the major clinical complication of peritoneal dialysis: the London, UK, peritonitis audit 2002-2003. Perit Dial Int 2009;29: 297–302.
59. Park SJ, Lee JY, Tak WT, et al. Using reagent strips for rapid diagnosis of peritonitis in peritoneal dialysis patients. Adv Perit Dial 2005;21:69–71.

60. Kofteridis DP, Valachis A, Perakis K, et al. Peritoneal dialysis-associated peritonitis: clinical features and predictors of outcome. Int J Infect Dis 2010;14: e489–93.

61. Jarvis EM, Hawley CM, McDonald SP, et al. Predictors, treatment, and outcomes of non-Pseudomonas Gram-negative peritonitis. Kidney Int 2010;78:408–14.

62. Fahim M, Hawley CM, McDonald SP, et al. Culture-negative peritonitis in peritoneal dialysis patients in Australia: predictors, treatment, and outcomes in 435 cases. Am J Kidney Dis 2010;55:690–7.

63. Restrepo C, Chacon J, Manjarres G. Fungal peritonitis in peritoneal dialysis patients: successful prophylaxis with fluconazole, as demonstrated by prospective randomized control trial. Perit Dial Int 2010;30:619–25.

64. Miles R, Hawley CM, McDonald SP, et al. Predictors and outcomes of fungal peritonitis in peritoneal dialysis patients. Kidney Int 2009;76:622–8.

65. Bunke CM, Brier ME, Golper TA. Outcomes of single organism peritonitis in peritoneal dialysis: gram negatives versus gram positives in the Network 9 Peritonitis Study. Kidney Int 1997;52:524–9.

66. Bunke M, Brier ME, Golper TA. Pseudomonas peritonitis in peritoneal dialysis patients: the Network #9 Peritonitis Study. Am J Kidney Dis 1995;25:769–74.

67. Smith TL, Pearson ML, Wilcox KR, et al. Emergence of vancomycin resistance in Staphylococcus aureus: glycopeptide-intermediate staphylococcus aureus Working Group. N Engl J Med 1999;340:493–501.

68. Piraino B, Bailie GR, Bernardini J, et al. Peritoneal dialysis-related infections recommendations: 2005 update. Perit Dial Int 2005;25:107–31.

69. Wiggins KJ, Johnson DW, Craig JC, et al. Treatment of peritoneal dialysis-associated peritonitis: a systematic review of randomized controlled trials. Am J Kidney Dis 2007;50:967–88.

70. de Vin F, Rutherford P, Faict D. Intraperitoneal administration of drugs in peritoneal dialysis patients: a review of compatibility and guidance for clinical use. Perit Dial Int 2009;29:5–15.

71. Chang TI, Kim HW, Park JT, et al. Early catheter removal improves patient survival in peritoneal dialysis patients with fungal peritonitis: results of ninety-four episodes of fungal peritonitis at a single center. Perit Dial Int 2011;31:60–6.

72. Posthuma N, Borgstein PJ, Eijsbouts Q, et al. Simultaneous peritoneal dialysis catheter insertion and removal in catheter-related infections without interruption of peritoneal dialysis. Nephrol Dial Transplant 1998;13:700–3.

73. Cancarini GC, Manili L, Brunori G, et al. Simultaneous catheter replacement-removal during infectious complications in peritoneal dialysis. Adv Perit Dial 1994;10:210–3.

74. Swartz RD, Messana JM. Simultaneous catheter removal and replacement in peritoneal dialysis infections: update and current recommendations. Adv Perit Dial 1999;15:205–8.

75. Chow KM, Szeto CC, Cheung KK, et al. Predictive value of dialysate cell counts in peritonitis complicating peritoneal dialysis. Clin J Am Soc Nephrol 2006;1: 768–73.

76. Kwan TH, Tong MK, Siu YP, et al. Ultrasonography in the management of exit site infections in peritoneal dialysis patients. Nephrology (Carlton) 2004;9: 348–52.

77. Szeto CC, Kwan BC, Chow KM, et al. Recurrent and relapsing peritonitis: causative organisms and response to treatment. Am J Kidney Dis 2009;54:702–10.

78. Aykut S, Caner C, Ozkan G, et al. Mupirocin application at the exit site in peritoneal dialysis patients: five years of experience. Ren Fail 2010;32:356–61.

79. Crabtree JH, Burchette RJ, Siddiqi RA, et al. The efficacy of silver-ion implanted catheters in reducing peritoneal dialysis-related infections. Perit Dial Int 2003;23: 368–74.

80. Prabhu MV, Subhramanyam SV, Gandhe S, et al. Prophylaxis against fungal peritonitis in CAPD—a single center experience with low-dose fluconazole. Ren Fail 2010;32:802–5.

Medical Device–Associated Infections in the Long-Term Care Setting

Christopher J. Crnich, MD, MS[a,b],*, Paul Drinka, MD[c,d,e]

KEYWORDS

- Device-related infection • Drug resistance • Long-term care
- Elderly • Geriatric

Long-term care facilities (LTCFs) are heterogeneous in size and the populations they serve. Although the number of LTCFs and bed capacity in the United States dropped by 9% and 13%, respectively, from the years 1999 to 2008, the overall number of individuals who spent at least some time in a LTCF actually increased from 3.09 million residents in 2004 to 3.27 million residents in 2008.[1] Economic forces driving reduced hospital length of stay have shifted an increasing amount of complex medical care to the ambulatory setting and skilled nursing facilities (SNF).[2] The resulting rise in the number of postacute residents in LTCFs has also increased use of indwelling medical devices in this setting. LTCF residents with indwelling medical devices have a significantly higher risk of developing a healthcare-associated infection (odds ratio [OR] 3.65; $P<0.001$)[3] and such devices have consistently been shown to be a risk factor for colonization or infection with multidrug-resistant bacteria, such methicillin-resistant *Staphylococcus aureus* (MRSA) and resistant gram-negative bacteria.[4–7] It is imperative that clinicians who practice in LTCFs have a comprehensive

Funding Support: Not applicable to the contents of this manuscript.

Conflicts of Interest: The authors have nothing to disclose.

[a] Division of Infectious Diseases, School of Medicine and Public Health, University of Wisconsin, 1685 Highland Avenue, 5217 MFCB, Madison, WI 53705, USA

[b] William S. Middleton Veterans Affairs Hospital, 2500 Overlook Terrace, Madison, WI 53705, USA

[c] Division of Geriatrics, School of Medicine and Public Health, University of Wisconsin, 1685 Highland Avenue, Madison, WI 53705, USA

[d] Division of Geriatrics, Medical College of Wisconsin, 8701 Watertown Plank Road, Milwaukee, WI 53226, USA

[e] Department of Internal Medicine, School of Medicine and Public Health, University of Wisconsin, Medical College of Wisconsin, 8701 Watertown Plank Road, Milwaukee, WI 53226, USA

* Corresponding author. Division of Infectious Diseases, School of Medicine and Public Health, University of Wisconsin, 1685 Highland Avenue, 5217 MFCB, Madison, WI 53705.

E-mail address: cjc@medicine.wisc.edu

Infect Dis Clin N Am 26 (2012) 143–164

doi:10.1016/j.idc.2011.09.007

0891-5520/12/$ – see front matter Published by Elsevier Inc.

understanding of the risks of infection associated with indwelling medical devices, the practices to reduce these risks, and the best way to intervene when prevention efforts fall short.

USE OF INVASIVE MEDICAL DEVICES IN LTCFs

An increasing variety of indwelling medical devices are encountered in LTCFs (**Box 1**). The most detailed data on the use of indwelling medical devices in LTCFs to date come from the Veterans Affairs (VA) Community Living Centers (CLCs).[3,8] In two system-wide point prevalence studies, Tsan and colleagues[3,8] found that approximately 25% of residents in VA CLCs had at least one invasive medical device (**Fig. 1**). Data on the use of indwelling medical devices in non-VA LTCFs are less comprehensive. Increasing external regulatory oversight[9] and public reporting of quality measures for SNFs has led to a reduction in the use of chronic urinary catheters and feeding tubes in long-term stay residents. For example, the proportion of long-term stay residents with a chronic urinary catheter decreased from 8.6% in 1991 to 4.8% by 2010.[10,11] Similarly, the prevalence of feeding tubes dropped from 4.4% in 1999 to 3.1% in 2008.[1] In contrast to the encouraging patterns seen in long-term stay residents, an increasing number of postacute-care residents are admitted to LTCFs with an indwelling medical device already in place. Approximately 12.6% of residents newly admitted to a LTCF were found to have an indwelling urinary catheter in a recent survey across five states[12] and the number of SNFs that provide infusion-related services has increased during the past decade resulting in an increased prevalence of intravascular catheters in this setting.

INFECTION OF INDWELLING URINARY CATHETERS
Use and Risk of Infection

Symptomatic urinary tract infection (UTI) is the second most common infectious complication encountered in LTCFs with reported incidence density rates ranging from 0.2 to 2.2 per 1000 resident-days.[13] Use of a urinary catheter is the predominant risk factor for UTI[14,15] and catheter-associated UTI (CAUTI) is the most common cause of bacteremia in LTCFs.[15,16] Studies performed before the current decade documented high rates, ranging from 7% to 12%, of chronic urinary catheter use in

---

Box 1
Types of invasive medical devices typically encountered in residents of LTCFs

Indwelling urinary device
    Urethral catheter
    Suprapubic catheter
Feeding tube
    Percutaneous endoscopic gastrostomy tube
    Nasogastric tube
Central venous catheter
    Peripherally inserted central venous catheter
    Cuffed and tunneled Hickman-like catheter
    Hemodialysis catheter
Tracheostomy tube

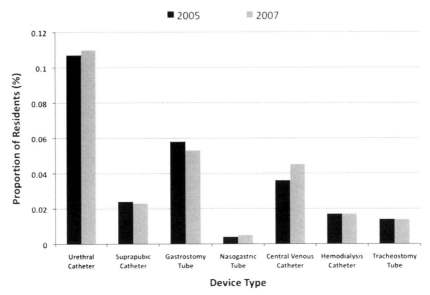

Fig. 1. Prevalence of different invasive medical devices among residents of Veterans Affairs Community Living Centers in 2005 and 2007, respectively. (*Data from* Tsan L, Davis C, Langberg R, et al. Prevalence of nursing home-associated infections in the Department of Veterans Affairs nursing home care units. Am J Infect Control 2008;36(3):173–9; and Tsan L, Langberg R, Davis C, et al. Nursing home-associated infections in Department of Veterans Affairs community living centers. Am J Infect Control 2010;38(6):461–6.)

LTCFs.[17,18] More recent data put the proportion of residents with a chronic urinary catheter at approximately 5%, although almost 13% of postacute care residents have a urinary catheter present at the time of admission to a LTCF.[12] Higher use rates are seen in VA CLCs where approximately 14% of residents either had an indwelling urethral or suprapubic urinary catheter during point prevalence surveys in 2005 and 2007.[3,8]

Pathogenesis

The pathogenesis of CAUTI is discussed in greater detail elsewhere in this issue. Briefly, organisms present on the periurethral mucosa may ascend to the bladder either on the outside of the catheter or may ascend on the inside of the catheter after contamination of the collecting system during manipulation by a healthcare worker (**Fig. 2**).[19] Bacterial introduction into the urinary tract occurs at a rate of 3% to 7% per day of catheterization, which means that bacteriuria is universal among residents catheterized for 30 days or more.[14] Once introduced, invading bacterial species uniformly reach high levels ($>10^5$ colony forming units) in the presence of an indwelling device[20] and often persist as they become incorporated into the biofilm that inevitably develops on the surface of the indwelling device.[21]

Diagnosis

Urine should always be sent for analysis and culture when considering antimicrobial treatment for suspected CAUTI. Ideally, this specimen should be obtained after placement of a new catheter to more accurately determine if recovered uropathogens localize to the bladder or are simply incorporated in the catheter biofilm.[14] Bacteriuria

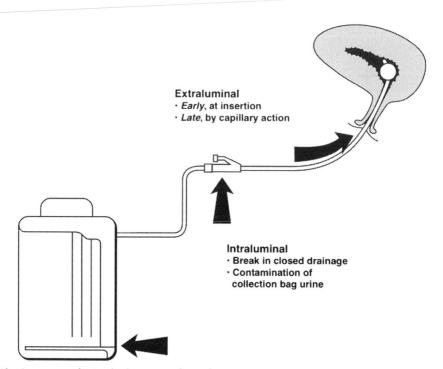

Fig. 2. Routes of microbial entry to the catheterized urinary tract. (*From* Juthani-Mehta M, Tinetti M, Perrelli E, et al. Diagnostic accuracy of criteria for urinary tract infection in a cohort of nursing home residents. J Am Geriatr Soc 2007;55(7):1072–7; with permission.)

is extremely prevalent in chronically catheterized individuals and most also have pyuria and elevations in urinary nitrites; therefore, an abnormal urinalysis or positive urine culture should never be used as the sole criteria for making a diagnosis of CAUTI (**Table 1**). Many cognitively impaired LTCF residents are unable to adequately articulate the presence of urinary symptoms and it is well-known that the fever response to infection can be attenuated in the elderly.[22,23] This has engendered the widespread belief that more subtle geriatric symptoms (eg, confusion, falls, or new urinary incontinence) are often the only manifestation of CAUTI in the LTCF setting.[24] However, there is no evidence that UTI is associated with the development of isolated geriatric symptoms,[25] nor is there any convincing published evidence that antimicrobial therapy leads to improvements in residents with bacteriuria and isolated geriatric symptoms.[26] The authors and others[27–29] believe it is important that at least one objective sign of infection (eg, evidence of systemic inflammation or localizing urinary signs or symptoms; see **Table 1**) be present before arbitrarily ascribing a resident's geriatric symptoms to CAUTI. Observation while awaiting the results of urine culture and pursuing alternative explanations for the change in condition is often warranted in residents with isolated geriatric manifestations of illness.

Treatment

Antimicrobial therapy of asymptomatic bacteriuria does not reduce the frequency of symptomatic infection and serves only to select for resistant uropathogens that make treatment of symptomatic infections more difficult.[30–32] For these reasons,

Table 1
Clinical signs and symptoms that may suggest the presence of a urinary tract infection[a] in catheterized long-term care facility residents

Signs of Systemic Inflammation	Localizing Symptoms	Nonlocalizing Symptoms
Fever[b]	Suprapubic tenderness	Acute change in mental status
Leukocytosis (white blood count $\geq$14,000 cells/mm^3 or >6% total band neutrophil count)	Costovertebral angle pain or tenderness	Acute change in functional status
Hypotension	Purulent discharge around catheter	New falls
	Acute pain, swelling, or tenderness of testes, epididymis, or prostate	Acute urinary incontinence
	New gross hematuria	

[a] Resident should have a positive urine culture or a urine culture pending before antibiotics are started.
[b] Defined as (1) a single temperature >37.8°C (100°F); (2) repeated temperature >37.2°C (99°F); or (3) a >1.1°C (2°F) increase in temperature from baseline.[22]

treatment of asymptomatic bacteriuria should be reserved for patients scheduled to undergo a urologic procedure.[14]

Patients with suspected CAUTI should have their urinary catheter changed before obtaining urinary cultures. This practice has also been shown to hasten the resolution of symptoms and reduce the frequency of 28-day relapse rates in at least one randomized trial.[33] Data on the optimal length of therapy for CAUTI and its attendant complications are limited. Current guidelines recommend that therapy for CAUTI be given for at least 7 days. Clinicians should consider the possibility of prostatitis, nephrolithiasis, or a perinephric abscess in residents whose symptoms are slow to respond despite appropriate coverage of organisms recovered from culture. In these cases, the antimicrobial therapy should be continued while additional diagnostic studies are explored.

Prevention

Guidelines for the prevention of CAUTI were recently updated by the Infectious Disease Society of America.[34] These guidelines appropriately emphasize limiting the use of indwelling urinary devices to well-defined clinical situations (**Table 2**). Notably, urinary incontinence is not considered an appropriate indication for chronic indwelling urinary catheterization unless there is a superimposed wound or palliative care need. With this more restrictive view of the appropriate use, as many as half of residents recently transferred from an acute-care facility do not qualify for continued catheterization.[35] It is imperative that LTCFs make expedited removal of unnecessary urinary devices a prominent component of any comprehensive CAUTI prevention program. To facilitate this objective, clinicians should consider the use of incontinence pads, intermittent urethral catheterization, or an external collecting device (eg, condom catheter) as alternatives.[34] Additional CAUTI prevention practices are detailed in **Box 2**.

Anti-infective catheters, which have been shown to reduce rates of bacteriuria in hospitalized patients with short-term urinary catheters,[19] have little role in patients with a chronic indwelling urinary catheter. Likewise, suppressive systemic antibiotics, urinary sterilizing agents (methenamine salts), or cranberry products, which may have situational applicability, have not been shown to reliably reduce the risk of CAUTI in the

Table 2
Appropriate indications for a chronic indwelling urinary catheter[a] in residents of a long-term care facility

Indication	Comment
Bladder outlet obstruction	When surgical correction is not considered feasible.
Neurogenic bladder with urinary retention	In residents with complete loss of bladder function who are unable to perform intermittent self-catheterization.
Urinary incontinence	As part of a comprehensive wound care plan in residents who have an open sacral or perineal wound or those individuals who have undergone select urologic or gynecologic surgery. In residents who are on hospice or comfort care who fail less invasive methods (eg, behavioral or pharmacologic, incontinence pads) and are not candidates for external collecting.

[a] Does not encompass appropriate indications for short-term urinary catheterization, such as management of acute urinary retention or monitoring of urinary output during aggressive diuresis or fluid challenge.

chronically catheterized patient and their routine use is discouraged in consensus guidelines.[19] The use of a suprapubic catheter rather than a urethral catheter has not convincingly been shown to reduce the risk of CAUTI but may be considered in the male resident with epididymitis or repeated urethral trauma with catheter exchanges or self-removal.

The well-known risk of catheter blockage from encrustations that form in the presence of urease-producing bacteria, such as *Proteus mirabilis*,[39] has given rise to two catheter management strategies of dubious benefit, at least with regard to the prevention of CAUTI. Routine irrigation of the catheterized bladder with saline,[40] antibiotics,[41] or antiseptic-containing solutions[42] has not been shown to reduce the frequency of obstruction or the risk of CAUTI in randomized trials. Similarly, routine replacement of the urinary catheter at a standard interval (every 2–4 weeks), which may reduce the risk of catheter obstruction,[43] has not clearly been shown to reduce CAUTI risk.[44] Admittedly, studies of this latter catheter maintenance practice are lacking. Future studies should strive to determine if there is true value to continuing this widely followed practice or whether it should go the way of other "standard practices" that were subsequently discarded after rigorous investigation.[45] Some experts advocate treatment of asymptomatic bacteriuria before urinary catheter exchange based on data demonstrating transient bacteremia and a higher incidence of fever among residents who have recently undergone placement of a urinary catheter.[46,47] However, there are no data that suggest that hard resident outcomes are improved by this practice and current guidelines discourage the routine use of antimicrobials with catheter exchange.[34]

INFECTION OF PERCUTANEOUS ENDOSCOPIC GASTROSTOMY TUBES

Since its introduction in the 1980,[48] placement of the percutaneous endoscopic gastrostomy (PEG) tube has become one the most widely performed medical procedures in the United States with an estimated 160,000 to 200,000 procedures performed annually.[49] PEG tubes may be placed using either a transoral or a transabdominal approach.[50] Although the cannulation success rate with either approach seems to

---

Box 2
Desirable components of a comprehensive program to prevent CAUTI in LTCFs

INSTITUTION-SPECIFIC URINARY CATHETER POLICIES AND PROCEDURES SHOULD BE DEVELOPED

Development of information systems that lead to actionable data:

1. Ongoing surveillance for catheter-associated urinary tract infections (per 1000 resident-days or 1000 catheter-days) using standard surveillance definitions[36] that are reported back to front-line staff on a regular basis

2. Audit and feedback of inappropriate urinary catheter use

3. Reorganization of the medical record to make prior antimicrobial history and urine culture results readily available to clinicians when a resident develops signs or symptoms consistent with[29,37]

4. Development of a facility-specific antibiogram of urinary isolates that is reviewed on a regular basis to identify resistance trends[37]

Clinical staff should receive education, training, and regular reinforcement of the following concepts and practices:

1. The appropriate indications for initiating urinary catheterization[38]

2. Proper aseptic technique when inserting a urinary catheter[34]

3. Proper catheter maintenance practices[34]:

    a. Hand hygiene and glove use whenever handing the urinary catheter or drainage system

    b. Keeping the urinary drainage bag below the level of the bladder at all times

    c. Properly secure indwelling catheters to prevent movement and urethral traction

    d. Minimizing handling and disconnections of the catheter from the drainage system

4. The importance of reassessing the continued need for a urinary catheter on a regular basis

Reduce unnecessary urinary catheterization through use of:

1. Checklists that provide clinicians with the appropriate indications for inserting a urinary catheter

2. Alternative methods for controlling urinary incontinence[34]

    a. Incontinence pads[14]

    b. Intermittent catheterization

    c. External drainage device[17]

3. A reminder system that prompts clinicians to evaluate the continued need for a urinary catheter in their residents

---

be equivalent, insertion by the transoral route remains the predominant method in the United States.

Use in LTCFs

The overall proportion of residents in LTCFs with a PEG tube is approximately 3.1% in non-VA LTCFs[1] and runs close to 5.5% in VA CLCs (see **Fig. 1**).[3,8] However, the prevalence of PEG tubes among LTCF residents with cognitive impairment is significantly higher. Approximately one-third of United States nursing home residents with advanced dementia undergo feeding tube placement[51] with an estimated incidence of 53.6 insertions per 1000 residents.[52]

Peristomal Wound Infections

Infectious complications after placement of a PEG tube occur most commonly within the month following insertion but can occur at any time. Most infections involve the peristomal skin, which complicates approximately 4% to 25% of insertions.[53] These infections usually are mild and typically manifest with localized pain, purulent drainage from around the tube, and erythema that extends outward from the insertion site. Systemic signs and symptoms, including fever and leukocytosis, are often absent and their presence, particularly when coupled with more severe or diffuse abdominal pain, should raise concern about the presence of an abscess, fasciitis, or peritonitis.

Although peristomal wound infections in patients with tubes placed by the transabdominal approach are typically caused by organisms of cutaneous origin, infections after tube insertion by the transoral approach derive from oropharyngeal organisms that contaminate the catheter during its transoral passage to the stomach.[54–56] Rates of peristomal wound infection seem to be significantly higher with the transoral rather than the transabdominal approach for PEG tube insertion.[57] Other features of the insertion and characteristics of the patient undergoing the procedure also seem to influence the risk of infection (**Table 3**).[58–60]

Clinicians treating a patient with a suspected peristomal wound infection should perform a careful physical examination to assess for the presence of a more complicated process (abscess, peritonitis, or necrotizing fasciitis) and to rule out the presence of a more benign process (dermatitis or superficial yeast infection) that does not require systemic antibiotics. It is recommended that a white cell blood count be obtained when evaluating fever and infection in the LTCF setting[61] and cultures of wound drainage should be sent based on published studies documenting high recovery rates of drug-resistant bacteria, such as MRSA and *Pseudomonas aeruginosa* (**Fig. 3**).[56–58,62–64] In patients with localized skin and soft tissue findings, it is reasonable to empirically start an oral agent that provides coverage for susceptible staphylococci, streptococci, and Enterobacteriaceae while awaiting culture. Patients with more severe manifestations, particularly those with systemic signs of illness, should be covered for MRSA and *P aeruginosa* pending the results of cultures. Most patients respond rapidly to oral agents, which should be given for 7 to 10 days. Complicated infections should be suspected in patients who present with significant systemic signs of infection or in those who fail to respond to oral therapy that has adequate activity against the organisms recovered from culture.

Table 3		
Factors associated with an elevated risk of developing a peristomal infection after placement of a percutaneous endoscopic gastrostomy tube		
Patient-Related Factors	**Procedure-Related Factors**	**Maintenance-Related Factors**
Diabetes mellitus	Placement by the transoral route rather than the "introducer" method	Excessive traction of the external bumper against the internal bumper
MRSA colonization	Failure to administer periprocedural antibiotics	Failure to use an external bumper
Obesity	Endoscopist inexperience	
Malnutrition	Use of a large caliber tube	
Corticosteroid use	Small abdominal wall incision	
Malignancy		

Abbreviation: MRSA, methicillin-resistant *Staphylococcus aureus*.

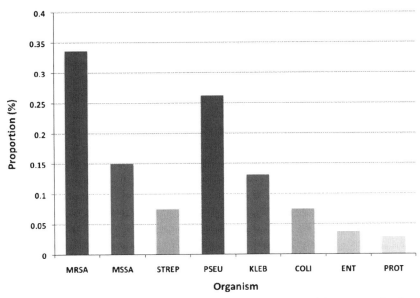

Fig. 3. The proportion of different microbial pathogens recovered from wound culture in patients diagnosed with peristomal wound infections. Data are derived from 107 microbiologically confirmed cases from six published studies. COLI, *Escherichia coli*; ENT, *Enterobacter* sp; KLEB, *Klebsiella* sp; MRSA, methicillin-resistant *Staphylococcus aureus*; MSSA, methicillin-sensitive *S aureus*; PROT, *Proteus mirabilis*; PSEU, *Pseudomonas aeruginosa*; STREP, *Streptococcus* sp. (*Data from* references.57–59, 62–64)

Complicated PEG Tube Infections

Serious infectious complications after PEG tube insertion are uncommon. Abscess at the insertion site has been described as a rare event (<1%) in most published series,[60,62,65] although one longitudinal study in a LTCF reported that 6 (10.3%) of 58 residents with a PEG tube developed an abscess at the insertion site during 4 years of follow-up.[66] When suspected, imaging with ultrasound or CT should be performed to confirm the presence of an abscess along with an aspiration to identify the causative pathogens. Most peristomal abscesses require surgical debridement or placement of a percutaneous drain, although small fluid collections can sometimes be managed conservatively with parenteral antimicrobials and repeat imaging.

Peritonitis occurs in 0.5% to 2% of PEG tube insertions in published series[67,68] and may occur early as a complication of insertion or later during tube dislodgements or reinsertions that are traumatic enough to disrupt the mature tract between the gastric and parietal peritoneal walls. A tube contrast imaging study is useful for determining if a disrupted tract or gastric leak is the cause of peritonitis. Surgical intervention is almost always required when disruption of the tract is documented.

Necrotizing fasciitis is an extremely rare complication associated with PEG tube placement.[69] It should be an early consideration in patients with systemic symptoms out of proportion to their local clinical examination and, when considered, should prompt abdominal imaging to identify air in the abdominal wall. Even with early and aggressive surgical debridement, mortality often exceeds 50%.[69]

Prevention

The use of cephalosporin-based prophylaxis at the time of transoral PEG tube insertion is now considered a standard of care and can reduce the risk of peristomal wound infection by nearly 70% compared with procedures in which no antibiotics are used (OR 0.31; 95% confidence interval, 0.22–0.44).[53] MRSA colonization has been identified as a significant risk factor for peristomal wound infection after PEG tub insertion.[59] Some centers have reported significant reductions in rates of infectious complications by screening and decolonizing patients before PEG tube insertion,[70,71] although this has not yet become a standard of care in published guidelines.[53] Using a protective sheath to minimize catheter contamination during transoral tube placement has also been shown to significantly reduce the risk of infection, but such a device is not yet commercially available in the United States.[72] Using the transabdominal approach for tube insertion seems to substantially reduce the risk of peristomal wound infection[57] but is not widely performed, perhaps because of perceptions of a higher risk of balloon rupture or deflation with the transabdominal catheters used in early studies.[73]

INFECTION OF INTRAVASCULAR DEVICES
Use

In the LTCF setting, most intravascular devices (IVDs) are intended for long-term (>10 days) rather than short-term use. Approximately 3.6% of the residents in VA CLCs had a long-term IVD present during a point-prevalence study performed in 2005[3] and a follow-up study found that use had increased to 4.5% by 2007.[8] The use of indwelling hemodialysis catheters was stable across the two surveillance periods (1.7%).[3,8] To the authors' knowledge, the extent of IVD use in non-VA LTCFs has not been reliably quantified. However, the continued expansion of postacute-care services in LTCFs in response to existing financial incentives[74] supports the notion that IVD use in these facilities is increasing.[75]

Risk and Pathogenesis of Infection

Prospective studies, in which every attempt was made to conclusively identify the presence of an IVD-related bloodstream infection (IVDR BSI), show that every type of IVD carries some risk, although the magnitude varies (**Table 4**).[76] Although host characteristics, such as critical illness, neutropenia, and AIDS, can modify the risk of IVDR BSI,[77,78] the characteristics of the IVD and the features of its insertion and maintenance seem to have a far greater impact on the overall risk of infection.[78]

Table 4
Rates of bloodstream infection associated with different types of long-term intravascular devices

Device Type	Rate per 1000 Device Days	
	Pooled Mean	95% CI
Peripherally inserted central catheters	1.0	0.8–1.2
Cuffed and tunneled Hickman-like catheters	1.6	1.5–1.7
Cuffed and tunneled hemodialysis catheters	1.6	1.5–1.7
Subcutaneous central venous ports	0.1	0.0–0.1

Data from Maki DG, Kluger DM, Crnich CJ. The risk of bloodstream infection in adults with different intravascular devices: a systematic review of 200 published prospective studies. Mayo Clin Proc 2006;81(9):1159–71.

For microorganisms to cause catheter-related infection they must first gain access to the extraluminal or intraluminal surface of the device where they can adhere, produce, and subsequently become incorporated into a biofilm that allows sustained infection and hematogenous dissemination.[79] Microorganisms may colonize an IVD by a variety of mechanisms (**Fig. 4**). With short-term devices, infection most commonly arises extraluminally as a result of bacterial colonization or infection at the skin insertion site.[78] In contrast, BSI associated with long-term IVDs, the type most commonly used in LTCFs, almost always arises intraluminally from contamination of the catheter hub and the luminal fluid.[80,81]

Microbiology

The microbial profile of IVDR BSI varies considerably based on the duration of catheterization (**Fig. 5**). Although gram-positive organisms cause nearly two-thirds of the microbiologically confirmed short-term IVD infections, these organisms are recovered in half of documented long-term IVD infections (see **Fig. 5**).[82] The opposite relationship is seen with the gram-negative bacteria, which cause 15% of the short-term IVD BSIs but more than a third of long-term infections (see **Fig. 5**).[82]

Diagnosis and Treatment

The diagnosis and treatment of IVDR BSI is discussed briefly. Infections associated with *S aureus* and gram-negative pathogens are typically abrupt in onset and patients almost always have signs of a systemic inflammatory response.[78] In contrast, IVDR BSI caused by coagulase-negative staphylococci and enterococci may manifest in a more indolent fashion. IVDR BSI should always be considered in the LTCF resident with a vascular catheter. Although current guidelines discourage their routine collection in LTCF residents with fever,[61] blood cultures, including one obtained from the

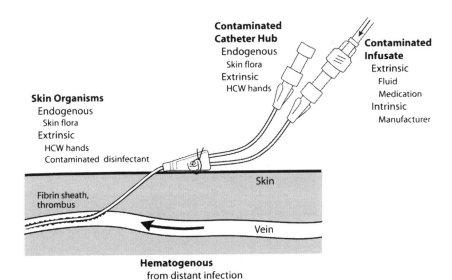

Fig. 4. The potential sources by which an intravascular device may become infected. HCW, healthcare worker. (*Adapted from* Crnich CJ, Maki DG. The promise of novel technology for the prevention of intravascular device-related bloodstream infection. I. Pathogenesis and short-term devices. Clin Infect Dis 2002;34(9):1232–42; with permission.)

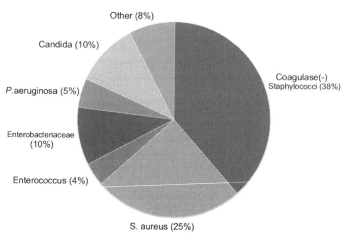

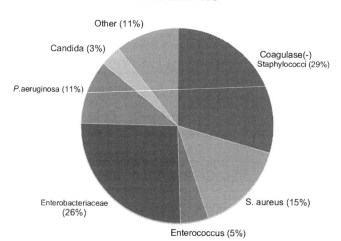

Fig. 5. Microbial pathogens recovered in patients with bloodstream infections associated with short- and long-term intravascular devices (IVDS). (*Data from* Maki DG, Kluger DM, Crnich CJ. Microbiology of intravascular device-related infection in adults: an analysis of 159 prospective studies and implications for treatment [abstract]. In: Proceedings and Abstracts of the 40th Annual Meeting of the Infectious Disease Society of America. Chicago: Infectious Disease Society of America; 2002.)

IVD and one from a peripheral vein, should always be obtained in the febrile resident who has a vascular catheter and no other localizing signs or symptoms.

Empiric antimicrobials that provide coverage for MRSA and *P aeruginosa* should be administered to residents with fever and systemic signs of inflammation and the catheter should be removed at the outset if there is evidence of a tunnel infection, thrombophlebitis, or severe sepsis.[78,83] Empiric antimicrobials may generally be withheld in otherwise clinically stable LTCF residents with isolated fever pending the results of blood cultures. Therapy should be targeted to the pathogens recovered after cultures have confirmed the diagnosis of IVDR BSI.

Prevention

The Centers for Disease Control and Prevention's Healthcare Infection Control Practices Advisory Committee and the Society for Healthcare Epidemiology of America have recently released evidence-based guidelines focused on the prevention of IVDR BSI.[84,85] Given the pathogenesis of infection with long-term IVDs, the primary focus for providers in LTCFs should be on minimizing contamination of the IVD hub and its luminal contents. LTCFs that provide infusion services should develop and regularly update their IVD maintenance policies and procedures. Similarly, facilities should ensure that staff members have received education and demonstrated their competency in IVD care and maintenance.

The basic foundation of preventing IVDR BSI rests with removing catheters when they are no longer needed and ensuring that providers adhere to recommended hygienic practices at all times. Specifically, it is important that LTCF staff always perform hand hygiene and wear clean or sterile gloves whenever handling the catheter or changing administration sets. Similarly, an appropriate antiseptic should always be used to swab the septum of the needless connector attached to the catheter whenever the port is being accessed. This is of particular importance, because suboptimal disinfection of needleless connectors before access has been linked to an increased risk of IVDR BSI.[86]

The use of novel technology to further reduce the risk of IVDR BSI has been an area of intense activity in recent years. Anti-infective lock solutions are the best studied of these technologies. A recently published meta-analysis found that vancomycin-containing lock solution reduced the risk of IVDR BSI by 66% (OR 0.34; 95% confidence interval, 0.12–0.98).[87] Similar benefits have been documented with other types of anti-infective lock solutions.[78] Nevertheless, none of these products have yet been commercialized and none are approved by the Food and Drug Administration for marketing. As a result, current guidelines recommend that anti-infective lock solutions be reserved only for individuals who have a history of recurrent IVDR BSI.[85]

The development of a needleless connector that is intrinsically resistant to bacterial colonization is another technology of considerable interest. Studies have shown that differences in connector design can influence the risk of internal surfaces becoming contaminated after a microbial challenge of the device.[88] Connectors impregnated with silver have been approved for commercial use; however, clinical trial data demonstrating their impact on risk of IVDR BSI are lacking. Paradoxically, the introduction of certain types of positive-pressure needleless connectors has been convincingly implicated as a cause of IVDR BSI in several hospitals and negative or neutral-pressure devices may pose a similar risk.[89] Whether these studies represent a problem that is specific to certain manufacturers or is suggestive of a problem that can be generalized to all mechanical needleless connectors is not clear. What is clear is that facilities need to perform a comprehensive product assessment before introducing new technology, and further reinforces the need for LTCFs that provide infusion services to develop and maintain a surveillance system for IVDR BSI.

INFECTION OF TRACHEOSTOMY DEVICES

Tracheostomy devices are placed for (1) relief of upper airway obstruction, most commonly caused by tumor or surgery; (2) access for suctioning and removal of airway secretions in individuals who cannot clear them on their own; or (3) provision of a stable airway in individuals who require prolonged mechanical ventilation.[90] Approximately 10% of hospitalized patients who require mechanical ventilation receive a tracheostomy[91] and rates of tracheostomy procedures in the United States have increased dramatically during the past 15 years.[92,93] Individuals with tracheostomy devices receive their care in a wide variety of institutional and ambulatory care settings; this section focuses on the infectious complications associated with the use of these devices in SNFs and long-term acute care (LTAC) facilities.

Use in LTCFs

Approximately 1.4% of residents in VA CLCs have a tracheostomy device (see **Fig. 1**), although most do not require mechanical ventilation.[3,8] A similar accounting of the use of tracheostomy devices in non-VA LTCFs is not readily available. However, in a recent study performed in North Carolina, the incidence rate of tracheostomy procedures in patients requiring prolonged mechanical ventilation increased 188% from the years 1993 to 2002.[92] Over half of these patients were discharged to a LTAC or rehabilitation facility. These data are consistent with studies from other states that have documented large increases in the number of individuals receiving posthospitalization mechanical ventilation in LTCFs.[94]

Clinical Presentation of Infection

Infection in patients with a tracheostomy device may manifest as either pneumonia or tracheobronchitis[95] and requires more than simply recovering a pathogen from culture because airway colonization is ubiquitous in this population.[95,96] Although some question whether tracheobronchitis exists in the ICU setting,[97] most authorities accept it as a real clinical entity among patients requiring chronic ventilatory support.[95]

The diagnosis of pneumonia in these patients should be based on a combination of cough; increasing purulent secretions; systemic signs of inflammation, such as fever and leukocytosis; impairments in gas exchange; localized auscultory findings; and the presence of an infiltrate on chest imaging. Patients with tracheobronchitis may present in a similar manner but do not typically have impairments in gas exchange and should not have localizing examination and imaging findings.

Incidence of Infection

Almost 50% to 60% of patients receiving prolonged ventilatory support develop pneumonia,[95] although the daily risk of infection is lower than among patients receiving ventilatory support in the ICU.[98] For example, in two recently published studies, the incidence density rate of pneumonia in patients receiving chronic ventilatory support in LTAC and spinal cord injury facilities was 1.67 and 1.74 per 1000 ventilator-days, respectively.[99,100] These numbers are similar to rates of pneumonia reported in patients receiving home ventilatory support[101] but are substantially lower than rates of pneumonia reported in acute care facilities.[102] Similar to studies performed in the intensive care unit (ICU) setting, impairments in neurologic function and duration of mechanical ventilation have been identified as consistent risk factors for pneumonia in patients requiring prolonged mechanical ventilation.[99,100]

The incidence of an early stomal infection in days after percutaneous trachesotomy ranges from 0% to 5% (mean, 2.3%) for percutaneous tracheostomy and 0% to 33% (mean, 10.7%) for open surgical tracheostomy.[103] Data on the rate of tracheobronchitis in patients with an established tracheostomy device are more limited. Niederman and coworkers[104] reported that 9 of 15 subjects with a tracheostomy residing in a local rehabilitation facility developed clinical evidence of tracheobronchitis and that risk of this complication seemed to be associated with chronic upper airway colonization with P aeruginosa. In a study of 39 nonhospitalized patients with a tracheostomy, 30 episodes of infection requiring antibiotic treatment (5 pneumonias and 25 episodes of tracheobronchitis) occurred during 1 year of follow-up.[96] Finally, Palmer and coworkers[105] reported that all of the seven chronically ventilated patients whom they followed for 6-months required treatment for tracheobronchitis; however, none developed pneumonia.

Treatment of Infection

Empiric antimicrobial therapy guided by local microbial patterns and the patient's prior culture results should be initiated in patients with systemic signs of infection after performing a thorough examination and sending respiratory specimens for culture. The authors recommend withholding empiric therapy from patients with isolated respiratory symptoms (increasing purulence of respiratory secretions) in the absence of impairments in gas exchange or systemic signs of illness. This subset of patients often improves with more aggressive pulmonary toilet. However, if symptoms progress, the culture results then allow the initiation of targeted therapy and avoid several days of unnecessarily broad coverage.

A detailed discussion of the therapy of pneumonia and tracheobronchitis is beyond the scope of this article. Monotherapy targeted against the pathogens recovered from culture is sufficient in most situations,[100] although combination therapy or the adjunctive use of aesolized agents may be necessary for particularly problematic multidrug-resistant organisms.[95,106] Airway eradication is almost impossible because of avid adherence of organisms to tracheobronchial cells[107] and their incorporation into the biofilm on the tracheostomy device.[108] The purpose of antimicrobial therapy is to facilitate the patient's return to their baseline status rather than sterilizing the respiratory tract. Whether replacement of the tracheostomy device during episodes of infection can accelerate the resolution of symptoms and reduce the frequency of recurrent infections is an unresolved issue and not routinely recommended. Further studies on the optimal treatment of pneumonia and tracheobronchitis in this population are warranted.

Prevention of Infection

Minimizing sedation and providing good oral care are cornerstones of pneumonia prevention in patients with an indwelling respiratory device. Patients with a chronic indwelling tracheostomy device should have an individualized treatment plan to address airway secretions and humidity because inadequate removal of secretions and failure to maintain adequate airway humidity can lead to insippation and mucosal injury that facilitates infection.[98] Staff providing respiratory care must be trained and educated in the appropriate handling of respiratory therapy equipment and be absolutely meticulous with hand hygiene and glove use during manipulation of the tracheostomy device.

Weaning and eventual decannulation have the greatest impact on reducing an individual patient's future risk of infection, although this is not feasible in many. Therapist-driven protocols have been shown to shorten the time taken to wean from the mechanical ventilator in the ICU setting, but a more individualized approach may be required in weaning patients after prolonged mechanical ventilation.[109]

Novel approaches for reducing the risk of tracheostomy infections have been explored on a limited basis. The topical application of polymyxin E–tobramycin paste to the tracheastoma seemed to reduce the risk of airway colonization and infection in one small nonrandomized study of children requiring long-term mechanical ventilation.[110] Similarly, the use of prophylactic aerosolized antibiotics has been shown to reduce the risk of ventilator-associated pneumonia in patients in the ICU[111] but, to the authors' knowledge, has not been studied in ventilated patients outside of the ICU setting. The high probability of resistance emerging with the anti-infectives used in both of these studies likely limits the clinical applicability of either approach.

158 Crnich & Drinka

SUMMARY

Clinicians in LTCFs are likely to continue to encounter an increasing array of patients with indwelling medical devices. Understanding the appropriate use and maintenance of these devices and working aggressively to remove them when no longer needed are key components of preventing infectious complications associated with indwelling medical devices.

REFERENCES

1. Centers for Medicare & Medicaid Services. Available at: https://www.cms.gov/CertificationandComplianc/Downloads/nursinghomedatacompendium_508.pdf. Accessed January 5, 2011.
2. Jarvis W. Infection control and changing health-care delivery systems. Emerging Infect Dis 2001;7(2):170–3.
3. Tsan L, Davis C, Langberg R, et al. Prevalence of nursing home-associated infections in the Department of Veterans Affairs nursing home care units. Am J Infect Control 2008;36(3):173–9.
4. Terpenning M, Bradley S, Wan J, et al. Colonization and infection with antibiotic-resistant bacteria in a long-term care facility. J Am Geriatr Soc 1994;42(10):1062–9.
5. Smith P, Seip C, Schaefer S, et al. Microbiologic survey of long-term care facilities. Am J Infect Control 2000;28(1):8–13.
6. Trick W, Weinstein R, Demarais P, et al. Colonization of skilled-care facility residents with antimicrobial-resistant pathogens. J Am Geriatr Soc 2001;49(3):270–6.
7. Mody L, Maheshwari S, Galecki A, et al. Indwelling device use and antibiotic resistance in nursing homes: identifying a high-risk group. J Am Geriatr Soc 2007;55(12):1921–6.
8. Tsan L, Langberg R, Davis C, et al. Nursing home-associated infections in Department of Veterans Affairs community living centers. Am J Infect Control 2010;38(6):461–6.
9. Newman DK. Urinary incontinence, catheters, and urinary tract infections: an overview of CMS tag F 315. Ostomy Wound Manage 2006;52(12):34–6, 38, 40–4.
10. Harrington C, Carrillo H, Thollaug SC, et al. Nursing Facilities, Staffing, Residents, and Facility Deficiencies, 1992 Through 1998. Report prepared for the U.S. Health Care Financing Administration and the Agency for Health Care Policy and Research. San Francisco (CA): University of California, Department of Social and Behavioral Sciences; 2000.
11. American Health Care Association Reimbursement and Research Department. Trends in publicly reported nursing facility quality measures, 2011. Available at: http://www.ahcancal.org/research_data/trends_statistics/Documents/trends_nursing_facilities_quality_measures.pdf. Accessed January 5, 2011.
12. Rogers MA, Mody L, Kaufman SR, et al. Use of urinary collection devices in skilled nursing facilities in five states. J Am Geriatr Soc 2008;56(5):854–61.
13. Strausbaugh LJ, Joseph CL. The burden of infection in long-term care. Infect Control Hosp Epidemiol 2000;21(10):674–9.
14. Nicolle L. The chronic indwelling catheter and urinary infection in long-term-care facility residents. Infect Control Hosp Epidemiol 2001;22(5):316–21.
15. Muder RR, Brennen C, Wagener MM, et al. Bacteremia in a long-term-care facility: a five-year prospective study of 163 consecutive episodes. Clin Infect Dis 1992;14(3):647–54.

16. Mylotte JM, Tayara A, Goodnough S. Epidemiology of bloodstream infection in nursing home residents: evaluation in a large cohort from multiple homes. Clin Infect Dis 2002;35(12):1484–90.

17. Hebel JR, Warren JW. The use of urethral, condom, and suprapubic catheters in aged nursing home patients. J Am Geriatr Soc 1990;38(7):777–84.

18. Kunin CM, Douthitt S, Dancing J, et al. The association between the use of urinary catheters and morbidity and mortality among elderly patients in nursing homes. Am J Epidemiol 1992;135(3):291–301.

19. Maki DG, Tambyah PA. Engineering out the risk for infection with urinary catheters. Emerging Infect Dis 2001;7(2):342–7.

20. Garibaldi RA, Mooney BR, Epstein BJ, et al. An evaluation of daily bacteriologic monitoring to identify preventable episodes of catheter-associated urinary tract infection. Infect Control 1982;3(6):466–70.

21. Nickel JC, Costerton JW, McLean RJ, et al. Bacterial biofilms: influence on the pathogenesis, diagnosis and treatment of urinary tract infections. J Antimicrob Chemother 1994;33(Suppl A):31–41.

22. Castle S, Yeh M, Toledo S, et al. Lowering the temperature criterion improves detection of infections in nursing home residents. Aging Immunol Infect Dis 1993;4:67–76.

23. Roghmann M, Warner J, Mackowiak P. The relationship between age and fever magnitude. Am J Med Sci 2001;322(2):68–70.

24. Juthani-Mehta M, Tinetti M, Perrelli E, et al. Diagnostic accuracy of criteria for urinary tract infection in a cohort of nursing home residents. J Am Geriatr Soc 2007;55(7):1072–7.

25. Boscia J, Kobasa W, Abrutyn E, et al. Lack of association between bacteriuria and symptoms in the elderly. Am J Med 1986;81(6):979–82.

26. Drinka P, Crnich C. Diagnostic accuracy of criteria for urinary tract infection in a cohort of nursing home residents. J Am Geriatr Soc 2008;56(2):376–7.

27. Loeb M, Bentley D, Bradley S, et al. Development of minimum criteria for the initiation of antibiotics in residents of long-term-care facilities: results of a consensus conference. Infect Control Hosp Epidemiol 2001;22(2):120–4.

28. Loeb M, Brazil K, Lohfeld L, et al. Optimizing antibiotics in residents of nursing homes: protocol of a randomized trial. BMC Health Serv Res 2002;2(1):17.

29. Crnich C, Drinka P. Treatment of bacteriuria in older adults: still room for improvement. J Am Med Dir Assoc 2008;9(8):542–4.

30. Alling B, Brandberg A, Seeberg S, et al. Effect of consecutive antibacterial therapy on bacteriuria in hospitalized geriatric patients. Scand J Infect Dis 1975;7(3):201–7.

31. Warren JW, Anthony WC, Hoopes JM, et al. Cephalexin for susceptible bacteriuria in afebrile, long-term catheterized patients. JAMA 1982;248(4):454–8.

32. Nicolle L, Mayhew W, Bryan L. Prospective randomized comparison of therapy and no therapy for asymptomatic bacteriuria in institutionalized elderly women. Am J Med 1987;83(1):27–33.

33. Raz R, Schiller D, Nicolle LE. Chronic indwelling catheter replacement before antimicrobial therapy for symptomatic urinary tract infection. J Urol 2000; 164(4):1254–8.

34. Hooton TM, Bradley SF, Cardenas DD, et al. Diagnosis, prevention, and treatment of catheter-associated urinary tract infection in adults: 2009 International Clinical Practice Guidelines from the Infectious Diseases Society of America. Clin Infect Dis 2010;50(5):625–63.

35. Cools HJ, Van der Meer JW. Restriction of long-term indwelling urethral catheterisation in the elderly. Br J Urol 1986;58(6):683–8.

36. McGeer A, Campbell B, Emori T, et al. Definitions of infection for surveillance in long-term care facilities. Am J Infect Control 1991;19(1):1–7.
37. Drinka P, Crnich C. An approach to endemic multi-drug-resistant bacteria in nursing homes. J Am Med Dir Assoc 2005;6(2):132–6.
38. Saint S, Lipsky BA. Preventing catheter-related bacteriuria: should we? Can we? How? Arch Intern Med 1999;159(8):800–8.
39. Mobley HL, Warren JW. Urease-positive bacteriuria and obstruction of long-term urinary catheters. J Clin Microbiol 1987;25(11):2216–7.
40. Muncie HL, Hoopes JM, Damron DJ, et al. Once-daily irrigation of long-term urethral catheters with normal saline. Lack of benefit. Arch Intern Med 1989;149(2):441–3.
41. Warren JW, Platt R, Thomas RJ, et al. Antibiotic irrigation and catheter-associated urinary-tract infections. N Engl J Med 1978;299(11):570–3.
42. Davies AJ, Desai HN, Turton S, et al. Does instillation of chlorhexidine into the bladder of catheterized geriatric patients help reduce bacteriuria? J Hosp Infect 1987;9(1):72–5.
43. Kunin CM, Chin QF, Chambers S. Indwelling urinary catheters in the elderly. Relation of "catheter life" to formation of encrustations in patients with and without blocked catheters. Am J Med 1987;82(3):405–11.
44. Drinka PJ. Complications of chronic indwelling urinary catheters. J Am Med Dir Assoc 2006;7(6):388–92.
45. Cook D, Randolph A, Kernerman P, et al. Central venous catheter replacement strategies: a systematic review of the literature. Crit Care Med 1997;25(8):1417–24.
46. Warren JW, Damron D, Tenney JH, et al. Fever, bacteremia, and death as complications of bacteriuria in women with long-term urethral catheters. J Infect Dis 1987;155(6):1151–8.
47. Jewes LA, Gillespie WA, Leadbetter A, et al. Bacteriuria and bacteraemia in patients with long-term indwelling catheters: a domiciliary study. J Med Microbiol 1988;26(1):61–5.
48. Gauderer MW, Ponsky JL, Izant RJ. Gastrostomy without laparotomy: a percutaneous endoscopic technique. J Pediatr Surg 1980;15(6):872–5.
49. Gauderer M. Twenty years of percutaneous endoscopic gastrostomy: origin and evolution of a concept and its expanded applications. Gastrointest Endosc 1999;50(6):879–83.
50. McClave SA, Chang W. Complications of enteral access. Gastrointest Endosc 2003;58(5):739–51.
51. Mitchell SL, Teno JM, Roy J, et al. Clinical and organizational factors associated with feeding tube use among nursing home residents with advanced cognitive impairment. JAMA 2003;290(1):73–80.
52. Kuo S, Rhodes RL, Mitchell SL, et al. Natural history of feeding-tube use in nursing home residents with advanced dementia. J Am Med Dir Assoc 2009;10(4):264–70.
53. Lipp A, Lusardi G. A systematic review of prophylactic antimicrobials in PEG placement. J Clin Nurs 2009;18(7):938–48.
54. Hull M, Beane A, Bowen J, et al. Methicillin-resistant Staphylococcus aureus infection of percutaneous endoscopic gastrostomy sites. Aliment Pharmacol Ther 2001;15(12):1883–8.
55. Faias S, Cravo M, Claro I, et al. High rate of percutaneous endoscopic gastrostomy site infections due to oropharyngeal colonization. Dig Dis Sci 2006;51(12):2384–8.
56. Chuang C, Hung K, Chen J, et al. Airway infection predisposes to peristomal infection after percutaneous endoscopic gastrostomy with high concordance between sputum and wound isolates. J Gastrointest Surg 2009;14(1):45–51.

57. Maetani I, Tada T, Ukita T, et al. PEG with introducer or pull method: a prospective randomized comparison. Gastrointest Endosc 2003;57(7):837–41.
58. Lee JH, Kim JJ, Kim YH, et al. Increased risk of peristomal wound infection after percutaneous endoscopic gastrostomy in patients with diabetes mellitus. Dig Liver Dis 2002;34(12):857–61.
59. Mainie I, Loughrey A, Watson J, et al. Percutaneous endoscopic gastrostomy sites infected by methicillin-resistant *Staphylococcus aureus*: impact on outcome. J Clin Gastroenterol 2006;40(4):297–300.
60. Zopf Y, Konturek P, Nuernberger A, et al. Local infection after placement of percutaneous endoscopic gastrostomy tubes: a prospective study evaluating risk factors. Can J Gastroenterol 2008;22(12):987–91.
61. High KP, Bradley SF, Gravenstein S, et al. Clinical practice guideline for the evaluation of fever and infection in older adult residents of long-term care facilities: 2008 update by the Infectious Diseases Society of America. Clin Infect Dis 2009; 48(2):149–71.
62. Jain NK, Larson DE, Schroeder KW, et al. Antibiotic prophylaxis for percutaneous endoscopic gastrostomy. A prospective, randomized, double-blind clinical trial. Ann Intern Med 1987;107(6):824–8.
63. Ahmad I, Mouncher A, Abdoolah A, et al. Antibiotic prophylaxis for percutaneous endoscopic gastrostomy–a prospective, randomised, double-blind trial. Aliment Pharmacol Ther 2003;18(2):209–15.
64. Saadeddin A, Freshwater DA, Fisher NC, et al. Antibiotic prophylaxis for percutaneous endoscopic gastrostomy for non-malignant conditions: a double-blind prospective randomized controlled trial. Aliment Pharmacol Ther 2005;22(6): 565–70.
65. Gossner L, Keymling J, Hahn EG, et al. Antibiotic prophylaxis in percutaneous endoscopic gastrostomy (PEG): a prospective randomized clinical trial. Endoscopy 1999;31(2):119–24.
66. Bourdel-Marchasson I, Dumas F, Pinganaud G, et al. Audit of percutaneous endoscopic gastrostomy in long-term enteral feeding in a nursing home. Int J Qual Health Care 1997;9(4):297–302.
67. Hogan RB, DeMarco DC, Hamilton JK, et al. Percutaneous endoscopic gastrostomy: to push or pull. A prospective randomized trial. Gastrointest Endosc 1986;32(4):253–8.
68. Foutch PG, Woods CA, Talbert GA, et al. A critical analysis of the Sacks-Vine gastrostomy tube: a review of 120 consecutive procedures. Am J Gastroenterol 1988;83(8):812–5.
69. MacLean AA, Miller G, Bamboat ZM, et al. Abdominal wall necrotizing fasciitis from dislodged percutaneous endoscopic gastrostomy tubes: a case series. Am Surg 2004;70(9):827–31.
70. Rao GG, Osman M, Johnson L, et al. Prevention of percutaneous endoscopic gastrostomy site infections caused by methicillin-resistant *Staphylococcus aureus*. J Hosp Infect 2004;58(1):81–3.
71. Horiuchi A, Nakayama Y, Kajiyama M, et al. Nasopharyngeal decolonization of methicillin-resistant *Staphylococcus aureus* can reduce PEG peristomal wound infection. Am J Gastroenterol 2006;101(2):274–7.
72. Suzuki Y, Urashima M, Ishibashi Y, et al. Covering the percutaneous endoscopic gastrostomy (PEG) tube prevents peristomal infection. World J Surg 2006;30(8): 1450–8.
73. Deitel M, Bendago M, Spratt EH, et al. Percutaneous endoscopic gastrostomy by the "pull" and "introducer" methods. Can J Surg 1988;31(2):102–4.

74. Clark P. Emergence of infection control surveillance in alternative health care settings. J Infus Nurs 2010;33(6):363–70.
75. Smith P, Bennett G, Bradley S, et al. SHEA/APIC guideline: infection prevention and control in the long-term care facility, July 2008. Infect Control Hosp Epidemiol 2008;29(9):785–814.
76. Maki DG, Kluger DM, Crnich CJ. The risk of bloodstream infection in adults with different intravascular devices: a systematic review of 200 published prospective studies. Mayo Clin Proc 2006;81(9):1159–71.
77. Safdar N, Maki DG. Risk of catheter-related bloodstream infection with peripherally inserted central venous catheters used in hospitalized patients. Chest 2005; 128(2):489–95.
78. Crnich CJ, Maki DG. Intravascular device infection. In: Carrico R, editor. 3rd edition, APIC text of infection control and epidemiology, vol. 1. Washington, DC: Association for Professionals in Infection Control and Epidemiology; 2009. p. 24.1–24.22.
79. Crnich CJ, Maki DG. The promise of novel technology for the prevention of intravascular device-related bloodstream infection. I. Pathogenesis and short-term devices. Clin Infect Dis 2002;34(9):1232–42.
80. Linares J, Sitges-Serra A, Garau J, et al. Pathogenesis of catheter sepsis: a prospective study with quantitative and semiquantitative cultures of catheter hub and segments. J Clin Microbiol 1985;21(3):357–60.
81. Raad I, Costerton W, Sabharwal U, et al. Ultrastructural analysis of indwelling vascular catheters: a quantitative relationship between luminal colonization and duration of placement. J Infect Dis 1993;168(2):400–7.
82. Maki DG, Kluger DM, Crnich CJ. Microbiology of intravascular device-related infection in adults: an analysis of 159 prospective studies and implications for treatment [abstract: 385]. In: Proceedings and Abstracts of the 40th Annual Meeting of the Infectious Disease Society of America. Chicago: Infectious Disease Society of America; 2002. p. 112.
83. Mermel LA, Allon M, Bouza E, et al. Clinical practice guidelines for the diagnosis and management of intravascular catheter-related infection: 2009 Update by the Infectious Diseases Society of America. Clin Infect Dis 2009;49(1):1–45.
84. Marschall J, Mermel LA, Classen D, et al. Strategies to prevent central line-associated bloodstream infections in acute care hospitals. Infect Control Hosp Epidemiol 2008;29(Suppl 1):S22–30.
85. O'Grady NP, Alexander M, Burns LA, et al. Guidelines for the prevention of intravascular catheter-related infections. Clin Infect Dis 2011;52(9):e162–93.
86. Cookson ST, Ihrig M, O'Mara EM, et al. Increased bloodstream infection rates in surgical patients associated with variation from recommended use and care following implementation of a needleless device. Infect Control Hosp Epidemiol 1998;19(1):23–7.
87. Safdar N, Maki D. Use of vancomycin-containing lock or flush solutions for prevention of bloodstream infection associated with central venous access devices: a meta-analysis of prospective, randomized trials. Clin Infect Dis 2006;43(4):474–84.
88. Yébenes JC, Delgado M, Sauca G, et al. Efficacy of three different valve systems of needle-free closed connectors in avoiding access of microorganisms to endovascular catheters after incorrect handling. Crit Care Med 2008;36(9):2558–61.
89. Jarvis WR, Murphy C, Hall KK, et al. Health care-associated bloodstream infections associated with negative- or positive-pressure or displacement mechanical valve needleless connectors. Clin Infect Dis 2009;49(12):1821–7.

90. Durbin CG. Tracheostomy: why, when, and how? Respir Care 2010;55(8): 1056–68.
91. Stelfox HT, Crimi C, Berra L, et al. Determinants of tracheostomy decannulation: an international survey. Crit Care 2008;12(1):R26.
92. Cox CE, Carson SS, Holmes GM, et al. Increase in tracheostomy for prolonged mechanical ventilation in North Carolina, 1993-2002. Crit Care Med 2004;32(11): 2219–26.
93. MacIntyre NR, Epstein SK, Carson S, et al. Management of patients requiring prolonged mechanical ventilation: report of a NAMDRC consensus conference. Chest 2005;128(6):3937–54.
94. Divo MJ, Murray S, Cortopassi F, et al. Prolonged mechanical ventilation in Massachusetts: the 2006 prevalence survey. Respir Care 2010;55(12): 1693–8.
95. Ahmed QA, Niederman MS. Respiratory infection in the chronically critically ill patient. Ventilator-associated pneumonia and tracheobronchitis. Clin Chest Med 2001;22(1):71–85.
96. Harlid R, Andersson G, Frostell CG, et al. Respiratory tract colonization and infection in patients with chronic tracheostomy. A one-year study in patients living at home. Am J Respir Crit Care Med 1996;154(1):124–9.
97. Torres A, Valencia M. Does ventilator-associated tracheobronchitis need antibiotic treatment? Crit Care 2005;9(3):255–6.
98. Wright SE, VanDahm K. Long-term care of the tracheostomy patient. Clin Chest Med 2003;24(3):473–87.
99. Walkey AJ, Reardon CC, Sulis CA, et al. Epidemiology of ventilator-associated pneumonia in a long-term acute care hospital. Infect Control Hosp Epidemiol 2009;30(4):319–24.
100. García-Leoni ME, Moreno S, García-Garrote F, et al. Ventilator-associated pneumonia in long-term ventilator-assisted individuals. Spinal Cord 2010;48(12): 876–80.
101. Chenoweth CE, Washer LL, Obeyesekera K, et al. Ventilator-associated pneumonia in the home care setting. Infect Control Hosp Epidemiol 2007;28(8): 910–5.
102. Edwards JR, Peterson KD, Mu Y, et al. National Healthcare Safety Network (NHSN) report: data summary for 2006 through 2008, issued December 2009. Am J Infect Control 2009;37(10):783–805.
103. Delaney A, Bagshaw SM, Nalos M. Percutaneous dilatational tracheostomy versus surgical tracheostomy in critically ill patients: a systematic review and meta-analysis. Crit Care 2006;10(2):R55.
104. Niederman MS, Ferranti RD, Zeigler A, et al. Respiratory infection complicating long-term tracheostomy. The implication of persistent gram-negative tracheobronchial colonization. Chest 1984;85(1):39–44.
105. Palmer LB, Donelan SV, Fox G, et al. Gastric flora in chronically mechanically ventilated patients. Relationship to upper and lower airway colonization. Am J Respir Crit Care Med 1995;151(4):1063–7.
106. Le J, Ashley ED, Neuhauser MM, et al. Consensus summary of aerosolized antimicrobial agents: application of guideline criteria. Insights from the Society of Infectious Diseases Pharmacists. Pharmacotherapy 2010;30(6): 562–84.
107. Niederman MS, Merrill WW, Ferranti RD, et al. Nutritional status and bacterial binding in the lower respiratory tract in patients with chronic tracheostomy. Ann Intern Med 1984;100(6):795–800.

108. Solomon DH, Wobb J, Buttaro BA, et al. Characterization of bacterial biofilms on tracheostomy tubes. Laryngoscope 2009;119(8):1633–8.
109. Scheinhorn DJ, Chao DC, Hassenpflug MS, et al. Post-ICU weaning from mechanical ventilation: the role of long-term facilities. Chest 2001;120(Suppl 6): 482S–4S.
110. Morar P, Makura Z, Jones A, et al. Topical antibiotics on tracheostoma prevents exogenous colonization and infection of lower airways in children. Chest 2000; 117(2):513–8.
111. Falagas ME, Siempos II, Bliziotis IA, et al. Administration of antibiotics via the respiratory tract for the prevention of ICU-acquired pneumonia: a meta-analysis of comparative trials. Crit Care 2006;10(4):R123.

Reuse of Medical Devices: Implications for Infection Control

Emily K. Shuman, MD[a], Carol E. Chenoweth, MD[a,b],*

KEYWORDS

• Medical • Device • Reuse • Single use

The US Food and Drug Administration (FDA) defines a medical device as an item that is recognized in the official National Formulary, is used to diagnose, treat, or prevent disease, and is not a drug.[1] Complex medical devices such as surgical instruments and endoscopes are multiuse devices designed to be used on multiple patients over a prolonged period of time. For such devices, there are clear guidelines for reprocessing and sterilization.[2,3] Issues with device contamination and disease transmission generally occur when these guidelines are not strictly followed.

Devices designated by manufacturers as single-use devices are intended to be used on a single patient for 1 procedure. Many single-use devices, including needles and syringes used for injection, are truly intended for single use. However, complex single-use devices that are frequently used in surgical, endoscopic, and intravascular procedures are often reused for economic reasons. In resource-limited settings throughout the developing world, reuse of single-use devices is especially common because of cost constraints. Reprocessing of single-use devices is often problematic because of the lack of standardized procedures, and adverse events related to device contamination or damage do occur. Such events can potentially offset any cost savings gained from reuse.

This review addresses issues associated with reuse of medical devices from an infection control standpoint, and also takes into account economic and ethical considerations. The primary focus is on the reuse of single-use devices because clearer standards exist for multiuse devices. The principles of reprocessing and sterilization are discussed briefly, and examples of outbreaks associated with contamination of medical devices are described. Finally, the reuse of medical devices in the developing

The authors have nothing to disclose.
a Division of Infectious Diseases, University of Michigan, 3119 Taubman Center, 1500 East Medical Center Drive, Ann Arbor, MI 48109-5378, USA
b Department of Infection Control and Epidemiology, University of Michigan, Ann Arbor, MI, USA
* Corresponding author. Division of Infectious Diseases, University of Michigan, 3119 Taubman Center, 1500 East Medical Center Drive, Ann Arbor, MI 48109-5378.
E-mail address: cchenow@umich.edu

Infect Dis Clin N Am 26 (2012) 165–172
doi:10.1016/j.idc.2011.09.010
0891-5520/12/$ – see front matter © 2012 Elsevier Inc. All rights reserved.

id.theclinics.com

world, with an emphasis on complex single-use devices such as pacemakers, is discussed.

REPROCESSING AND STERILIZATION OF MEDICAL DEVICES

Critical medical devices enter sterile tissue or the vascular system.[2,4] Examples of critical devices include surgical instruments and catheters used for intravascular procedures such as cardiac catheterization. These devices must be sterilized between uses because any contamination with microorganisms can result in disease transmission. Sterilization is a process that destroys all microorganisms or spores. The method of sterilization (steam, gas, or chemical) depends on the heat and chemical sensitivity of the device. The methods for sterilization of various medical devices are well described.[2,4] The sterilization of prion-contaminated medical devices represents a special case because prions are not destroyed by standard sterilization methods. Critical devices that may be prion contaminated should be sterilized using the protocol summarized by Rutala and Weber.[4] Some critical devices are designated as single-use devices but are frequently reused (eg, catheters used for coronary angiography and electrophysiology procedures).

Semicritical medical devices come in contact with mucous membranes or nonintact skin but do not enter normally sterile tissues.[4] Examples include respiratory therapy and anesthesia equipment as well as endoscopes. Such devices do not require sterilization but should be reprocessed such that they are free of microorganisms (but not necessarily spores). High-level chemical disinfection is generally recommended for devices such as endoscopes, with the choice of specific disinfectant to be based on compatibility with the device.[2,3] High-level disinfection using heat rather than a chemical disinfectant is appropriate for devices such as respiratory therapy equipment.[4]

Noncritical medical devices come in contact with intact skin only.[4] Examples include blood pressure cuffs, bedpans, and other items frequently found in patients' hospital rooms. Transmission of microorganisms via noncritical devices most commonly occurs when the devices become contaminated with microorganisms from the hands of health care workers. Therefore, routine intermediate-level disinfection (removes most, but not all, microorganisms) or low-level disinfection (removes most microorganisms except for some mycobacteria and viruses) of noncritical devices is recommended.[2,4]

GUIDANCE FOR REUSE OF SINGLE-USE DEVICES

A single-use medical device is designated by the manufacturer as being indicated for single use on a single patient during 1 procedure.[1] Before the 1970s, most medical devices were made of glass and metal and were routinely reused. The development of single-use devices occurred because of the increasing use of new plastic materials and market demand for disposable devices.[1] However, after the introduction of single-use devices, many hospitals began reprocessing and reusing these devices to save money and reduce waste. In addition, because of the burden of reprocessing such devices, many hospitals began to outsource reprocessing to third parties.

During the 1990s, the FDA began to examine potential safety issues associated with the reuse of single-use devices. Between 1996 and 1999, 245 adverse events (7 deaths, 72 injuries, 147 device malfunctions, and 19 events classified as "other") related to the reuse of single-use devices were reported by manufacturers.[1] This pattern was not particularly different from that reported for the initial use of single-use devices but did prompt the FDA to examine the potential impact of the reprocessing and reuse of single-use devices under experimental conditions. These experiments showed that reprocessing resulted in the persistence of biofilms and degradation of materials, which could lead to transmission of infection and equipment failure.[1]

In 2000, the FDA released guidance regarding reprocessing and reuse of single-use devices for manufacturers, hospitals, and third-party reprocessing facilities.[1] This guidance allows the involved parties to assess the potential risk associated with device reuse. Risk assessment is partly based on the potential for transmission of infection, which takes into account both the intended use of the device (ie, whether it is critical, semicritical, or noncritical) and the presence of features that could impede adequate sterilization or disinfection. For example, devices such as catheters for intravascular procedures may have narrow lumens or interlocking parts in which debris may be retained. Risk assessment is also based on the potential for reprocessing to result in inadequate device performance. This assessment is largely based on postmarketing surveillance for a particular device as well as consensus performance standards, which may not be available for all devices. Based on overall risk assessment, for which algorithms are available from the FDA,[1] the risk of reprocessing and reuse of single-use medical devices may be classified as high, moderate, or low. Examples of commonly reused single-use devices along with their associated risk categories are provided in **Table 1**. The FDA guidance applies only to nonimplantable devices.

INFECTION CONTROL ISSUES RELATED TO THE REUSE OF MEDICAL DEVICES

There have been many outbreaks of infection associated with the reuse of medical devices, involving a variety of microorganisms including bacteria, mycobacteria, fungi, and viruses. Outbreaks have occurred in multiple settings, including after inappropriate reuse of single-use devices and after reuse of both single-use and multiuse devices that have been improperly sterilized or reprocessed. Examples of each setting follow.

There are many single-use devices that are truly intended for single use. For example, needles and syringes used for injection should be disposed of after 1 use and certainly should not be reused on other patients. However, in particular settings such as the developing world, these items are frequently reused. In a study of immunization practices in Africa, 15% to 60% of clinics reported reusing needles and syringes without sterilization, resulting in a large incidence of injection site abscesses.[5] Up to 55% of health care workers in rural Northwestern China reported reusing needles and syringes, and the number of children in China estimated to have acquired hepatitis B infection through unsafe vaccination practices is 135 to 3120 per 100,000 population.[6]

In 2008, the World Health Organization (WHO) estimated that unsafe medical injections resulted in 340,000 human immunodeficiency virus (HIV) infections, 15 million hepatitis B infections, 1 million hepatitis C infections, and 850,000 injection site abscesses worldwide.[7] Overall, transmission via unsafe injection practices accounted for 14% of HIV infections, 25% of hepatitis B infections, and 8% of hepatitis C infections. Although these numbers seem extraordinarily high, they represent a significant decrease in the number of infections since 2000, when the WHO established the Safe Injection Global Network (SIGN), which works with local communities to establish safe injection practices. Because of the SIGN program, it is estimated that 430,000 HIV infections, 5 million hepatitis B infections, and 1 million hepatitis C infections have been prevented in the developing world each year.[7]

Reuse of syringes with concomitant transmission of infection is not restricted to limited resource settings. In 2001, an outbreak of hepatitis C occurred at a

Table 1 Commonly reused single-use medical devices and their associated risk categories based on guidance from the FDA	
Device	**Risk Category**
Cardiovascular	
Catheters used for percutaneous transluminal coronary angioplasty and electrophysiology procedures	High
Blood pressure cuff	Low
Cardiac guidewire	High
Intra-aortic balloon catheter	High
Respiratory	
Breathing mouthpiece	Low
Endotracheal tube	High
Respiratory therapy and anesthesia breathing circuits	Moderate
Tracheobronchial suction catheter	High
Gastrointestinal/urologic	
Endoscopic guidewire	Low
Biopsy forceps	High
Urethral catheter	Moderate
Nephrology	
Hemodialysis blood tubing	Moderate
Orthopedics	
External fixation device	Low
Saw blades	Low
Surgical drills	Low
Surgery	
Electrosurgical electrodes and pencils	Moderate
Laparoscopic scissors	High
Dental	
Orthodontic braces	High

Data from Food and Drug Administration. Medical devices 2011. Available at: http://www.fda.gov/ MedicalDevices/default.htm. Accessed April 12, 2011.

hematology/oncology clinic in the United States.[8] In this outbreak, syringes used to draw blood were reused to draw saline flushes from shared saline bags. Another outbreak of hepatitis C occurred at an endoscopy center in Nevada because of the reuse of syringes and single-dose medication vials on multiple patients.[9] An outbreak of *Klebsiella pneumoniae* and *Enterobacter aerogenes* bloodstream infection occurred in a pain management clinic in New York City because of the reuse of single-dose vials for steroid injections on multiple patients.[10] Many other outbreaks of bloodborne pathogens have also been associated with reuse of multidose vials on multiple patients.[11] Outbreaks of bloodstream infection have also been reported with reuse of multiuse devices such as hemodialysis equipment, which is complex in design and can be difficult to disinfect.[12–14]

Reuse of single-use anesthesia and respiratory therapy equipment is common in the United States; this practice has been associated with outbreaks when appropriate reprocessing is not performed. An outbreak of respiratory tract infection due to *Bacillus cereus* occurred in a neonatal intensive care unit as a result of contamination of ventilator circuits.[15] In this outbreak, the hospital's low-temperature steam disinfector was broken, and reprocessing of equipment was outsourced to a third party. Similarly, an outbreak of respiratory tract colonization and infection due to *Burkholderia cepacia* was attributed to contamination of ventilator temperature probe tips.[14] Both true outbreaks and pseudo-outbreaks of *Pseudomonas aeruginosa* have occurred because of improper reprocessing of bronchoscopes, which are multiuse devices.[16,17]

There is heightened concern for potential risk of infection with reuse of complex single-use devices such as cardiac catheters. However, a study comparing infection risk in patients undergoing cardiac catheterization with disposable versus reprocessed catheters found that no patient developed infection.[18] Similarly, in a survey of 12 large medical centers, reuse of pacing catheters was common and was not associated with postprocedure infections.[19] In addition, there were no reported concerns regarding equipment failure due to reprocessing in either study.

ECONOMIC AND ETHICAL CONSIDERATIONS FOR REUSE OF SINGLE-USE DEVICES

Two Canadian studies have systematically examined economic considerations in the reuse of single-use medical devices. Hailey and colleagues[20] reviewed the literature and found that there was insufficient evidence to suggest that reuse of single-use devices is cost-effective. For example, the investigators found that eliminating the reuse of single-use devices for procedures such as laparoscopic cholecystectomy and coronary angioplasty would add less than 0.1% to the total cost for these procedures during the course of a year. Similarly, Jacobs and colleagues[21] found insufficient evidence to support reuse of single-use devices from an economic perspective, primarily because of lack of quality research. Only 9 articles met the investigators' search criteria, and they were all published before 2000. Although reuse of single-use devices resulted in 49% cost savings, the investigators noted that these savings could easily be offset by adverse events.

Because adverse events related to reuse of single-use devices are not often reported, data regarding outcomes are very limited, and it is often difficult to attribute adverse events to device reuse. A survey of Canadian hospitals that reprocess single-use devices found that 40% do not have a written policy regarding reprocessing, and 12% do not even have a mechanism by which to report potential adverse events.[20] In Brazil, where 97% of institutions responding to a survey reported reusing single-use devices for hemodynamic procedures, one-third of hospitals reported having no surveillance system for adverse events.[22] Only 22% reported using a standard reprocessing protocol.

The lack of data regarding outcomes associated with reuse of single-use devices raises important legal and ethical concerns. The FDA holds manufacturers and reprocessors (including third-party reprocessors) responsible for adverse events that occur as a result of reuse of single-use devices, which is considered to represent "remanufacturing" of the device.[1] Currently, it is not common practice to inform patients before procedures that a reprocessed device may be used. In the absence of adequate data regarding adverse outcomes associated with the reuse of single-use devices, it is difficult to advise patients appropriately about potential risks. Whereas most risks (eg, bleeding, risks associated with anesthesia) related to a procedure are more well-established, the risks associated with device reuse are largely hypothetical. Clinicians have a duty to report when an adverse event related to a device may have occurred, but there is little obligation to inform about such potential adverse events in advance.[20] The rules could change in the event of a high-level legal case concerning an adverse event related to single-use device reuse.

REUSE OF COMPLEX SINGLE-USE MEDICAL DEVICES IN RESOURCE-LIMITED SETTINGS

Reuse of single-use devices is common in resource-limited settings because of cost constraints. Unfortunately, inappropriate reuse of single-use devices such as needles and syringes frequently results in transmission of disease in developing countries. However, in more developed nations, reuse of complex medical devices that are not frequently reused has the potential to provide great benefit. The reuse of pacemakers is discussed here as an example.

Because of the expense involved, the use of pacemakers to treat symptomatic bradyarrhythmias in developing countries is virtually nonexistent. Recently, there has been an interest in postmortem pacemaker reuse for patients who would otherwise not have access to pacemaker therapy. Baman and colleagues[23] advocate a collaborative approach involving patients, funeral directors, physicians, and nonprofit charitable organizations to set up programs for pacemaker reutilization. The investigators propose a protocol for ensuring adequate functionality and sterilization of devices before reimplantation. Pilot programs have shown the feasibility of such an initiative. In addition, large surveys of patients with pacemakers have shown that most patients are willing to have their pacemakers removed for reuse after death.[24] Funeral directors have also expressed a willingness to cooperate with pacemaker removal and donation.[24] Furthermore, a large meta-analysis of 18 studies including 2270 patients with reprocessed pacemakers showed rates of device malfunction and infection that were no different from those for initial device implantation.[25] A major obstacle for implementation of pacemaker donation programs could be acceptance of used devices by potential recipients, although acceptance has been good in pilot programs. In addition, there are potential legal concerns due to FDA regulations on interstate commerce of medical devices, which are addressed by Baman and colleagues[23] in their proposal.

SUMMARY

Reuse of both single-use and multiuse medical devices occurs frequently. For many devices that are commonly reused, clear protocols for reprocessing and sterilization exist. However, for many single-use devices, such protocols do not exist, and institutions that reprocess such devices may not even have their own internal protocols. Because of the lack of high-quality data, it is not clear whether reuse of single-use devices provides significant economic benefit to health care facilities. Cost savings may occur, but the degree to which savings are offset by adverse events is uncertain. More research is needed to help answer these important questions. In addition, there are many potential legal and ethical issues related to the reuse of single-use devices, again stemming from the lack of standards and data regarding adverse events. Medical devices are commonly reused in developing countries because of cost constraints, sometimes inappropriately in the case of needle and syringe reuse for administration of vaccines. However, reuse of complex expensive medical devices such as pacemakers has the potential to provide great benefit in resource-limited settings as long as strict protocols are followed to avoid device malfunction and infection.

REFERENCES

1. Food and Drug Administration. Medical devices, 2011. Available at: http://www.fda.gov/MedicalDevices/default.htm. Accessed April 12, 2011.
2. Rutala WA, Weber DJ, Healthcare Infection Control Practices Advisory Committee. Guideline for disinfection and sterilization in healthcare facilities.

2008. Available at: http://www.cdc.gov/ncidod/dhqp/pdf/guidelines/Disinfection_Nov_2008.pdf. Accessed April 12, 2011.

3. Nelson DB, Jarvis WR, Rutala WA, et al. Multi-society guideline for reprocessing flexible gastrointestinal endoscopes. Society for Healthcare Epidemiology of America. Infect Control Hosp Epidemiol 2003;24(7):532–7.

4. Rutala WA, Weber DJ. Disinfection and sterilization in healthcare facilities. In: Lautenbach E, Woeltje KF, Malani PN, editors. Practical healthcare epidemiology. 3rd edition. Chicago: University of Chicago Press; 2010. p. 61–80.

5. Dicko M, Oni AQ, Ganivet S, et al. Safety of immunization injections in Africa: not simply a problem of logistics. Bull World Health Organ 2000;78(2):163–9.

6. Murakami H, Kobayashi M, Zhu X, et al. Risk of transmission of hepatitis B virus through childhood immunization in northwestern China. Soc Sci Med 2003;57(10):1821–32.

7. World Health Organization. SIGN meeting report, 2010. Available at: http://www.who.int/injection_safety/toolbox/sign2010_meeting.pdf. Accessed May 24, 2011.

8. Macedo de Oliveira A, White KL, Leschinsky DP, et al. An outbreak of hepatitis C virus infections among outpatients at a hematology/oncology clinic. Ann Intern Med 2005;142(11):898–902.

9. Centers for Disease Control (CDC). Acute hepatitis C virus infections attributed to unsafe injection practices at an endoscopy clinic—Nevada, 2007. MMWR Morb Mortal Wkly Rep 2008;57(19):513–7.

10. Wong MR, Del Rosso P, Heine L, et al. An outbreak of Klebsiella pneumoniae and Enterobacter aerogenes bacteremia after interventional pain management procedures, New York City, 2008. Reg Anesth Pain Med 2010;35(6):496–9.

11. Germain JM, Carbonne A, Thiers V, et al. Patient-to-patient transmission of hepatitis C virus through the use of multidose vials during general anesthesia. Infect Control Hosp Epidemiol 2005;26(9):789–92.

12. Centers for Disease Control (CDC). Bacteremia associated with reuse of disposable hollow-fiber hemodialyzers. MMWR Morb Mortal Wkly Rep 1986;35(25):417–8.

13. Vanholder R, Vanhaecke E, Ringoir S. Pseudomonas septicemia due to deficient disinfectant mixing during reuse. Int J Artif Organs 1992;15(1):19–24.

14. Weems JJ Jr. Nosocomial outbreak of Pseudomonas cepacia associated with contamination of reusable electronic ventilator temperature probes. Infect Control Hosp Epidemiol 1993;14(10):583–6.

15. Gray J, George RH, Durbin GM, et al. An outbreak of Bacillus cereus respiratory tract infections on a neonatal unit due to contaminated ventilator circuits. J Hosp Infect 1999;41(1):19–22.

16. Silva CV, Magalhaes VD, Pereira CR, et al. Pseudo-outbreak of Pseudomonas aeruginosa and Serratia marcescens related to bronchoscopes. Infect Control Hosp Epidemiol 2003;24(3):195–7.

17. Shimono N, Takuma T, Tsuchimochi N, et al. An outbreak of Pseudomonas aeruginosa infections following thoracic surgeries occurring via the contamination of bronchoscopes and an automatic endoscope reprocessor. J Infect Chemother 2008;14(6):418–23.

18. Frank U, Herz L, Daschner FD. Infection risk of cardiac catheterization and arterial angiography with single and multiple use disposable catheters. Clin Cardiol 1988;11(11):785–7.

19. O'Donoghue S, Platia EV. Reuse of pacing catheters: a survey of safety and efficacy. Pacing Clin Electrophysiol 1988;11(9):1279–80.

20. Hailey D, Jacobs PD, Ries NM, et al. Reuse of single use medical devices in Canada: clinical and economic outcomes, legal and ethical issues, and current hospital practice. Int J Technol Assess Health Care 2008;24(4):430–6.
21. Jacobs P, Polisena J, Hailey D, et al. Economic analysis of reprocessing single-use medical devices: a systematic literature review. Infect Control Hosp Epidemiol 2008;29(4):297–301.
22. Amarante JM, Toscano CM, Pearson ML, et al. Reprocessing and reuse of single-use medical devices used during hemodynamic procedures in Brazil: a widespread and largely overlooked problem. Infect Control Hosp Epidemiol 2008; 29(9):854–8.
23. Baman TS, Kirkpatrick JN, Romero J, et al. Pacemaker reuse: an initiative to alleviate the burden of symptomatic bradyarrhythmia in impoverished nations around the world. Circulation 2010;122(16):1649–56.
24. Gakenheimer L, Lange DC, Romero J, et al. Societal views of pacemaker reutilization for those with untreated symptomatic bradycardia in underserved nations. J Interv Card Electrophysiol 2011;30(3):261–6.
25. Baman TS, Meier P, Romero J, et al. Safety of pacemaker reutilization: a meta-analysis with implications for underserved nations. Circ Arrhythm Electrophysiol 2011;4(3):318–23.

Novel Approaches to the Diagnosis, Prevention, and Treatment of Medical Device-Associated Infections

Paschalis Vergidis, MD[a], Robin Patel, MD[a,b],*

KEYWORDS

- Biofilm • Medical device
- Catheter-associated urinary tract infection
- Catheter-associated bloodstream infection
- Orthopedic implant infection
- Cardiovascular implantable electronic device infection

Indwelling devices are increasingly used in many areas of medical practice. The pathogenesis of device-associated infections relates to bacteria that attach to and grow on surfaces in complex communities. Microbial biofilms develop when microorganisms adhere to a surface and produce extracellular polymers that facilitate adhesion and provide a structural matrix. In addition to structural features, such biofilm bacteria exhibit distinct characteristics with respect to growth rate and protection from host immune mechanisms and antimicrobial agents.

Funding support: This publication was made possible by Grant Numbers R01 AR056647 and R01 AI091594 from the National Institute of Arthritis and Musculoskeletal and Skin Diseases, and the National Institute of Allergy and Infectious Diseases, respectively (National Institutes of Health).

Financial disclosure: Dr Patel has an unlicensed US patent pending for a method and an apparatus for sonication (and has forgone her right to receive royalties in the event that the patent is licensed). Dr Vergidis has nothing to disclose.

[a] Division of Clinical Microbiology, Department of Laboratory Medicine and Pathology, Mayo Clinic, 200 First Street Southwest, Rochester, MN 55905, USA

[b] Division of Infectious Diseases, Department of Internal Medicine, Mayo Clinic, 200 First Street Southwest, Rochester, MN 55905, USA

* Corresponding author. Division of Clinical Microbiology, Department of Laboratory Medicine and Pathology, Mayo Clinic 200 First Street Southwest, Rochester, MN 55905.

E-mail address: patel.robin@mayo.edu

Infect Dis Clin N Am 26 (2012) 173–186
doi:10.1016/j.idc.2011.09.012
0891-5520/12/$ – see front matter © 2012 Elsevier Inc. All rights reserved.

id.theclinics.com

Biofilm bacteria are up to 1000-fold more resistant to antimicrobial agents compared with planktonic bacteria, their free-living counterparts. An altered microenvironment, decreased growth rate with persister cells (a protected phenotypic state), antimicrobial-destroying enzymes within the matrix, quorum-sensing signaling systems that coordinate biological activity, and upregulation of stress-response genes are among the proposed mechanisms of reduced antimicrobial susceptibility.[1] Surgical implantation of a foreign body leads to tissue damage and consequently to an inflammatory response that enhances bacterial colonization. Chemical and physical properties of the foreign body also influence bacterial adherence. In addition to the innate antimicrobial resistance associated with the biofilm state, in the highly dense bacterial population within a biofilm, horizontal transfer of antimicrobial resistance genes can occur.

This article reviews innovative concepts for the prevention of biofilm formation and biofilm-directed therapeutics. The authors also discuss novel approaches for the diagnosis and prevention of catheter-associated urinary tract and bloodstream infections, and infections associated with orthopedic implants and cardiovascular implantable electronic devices (CIEDs).

PREVENTION OF BIOFILM FORMATION

A potential approach to prevent biofilm formation (and consequently device-associated infection) is the use of antisense molecules that silence bacterial genes responsible for virulence.[2] Due to their chemical stability, peptide nucleic acids are potential therapeutic candidates. Genes encoding bacterial factors responsible for adhesion and biofilm formation are potential targets for an antisense strategy. Such targets include a family of adhesins called Microbial Surface Components Recognizing Matrix Molecules (MSCRAMMs) that mediate bacterial adhesion to biomaterials,[3] and the *ica* locus, which harbors genes for production of polysaccharide intercellular adhesin, a component of the extracellular matrix of many staphylococcal biofilms.[4] To date, attempts at silencing adhesin genes have not been successful.

Another prevention strategy is based on interference with bacterial cell-to-cell communication using quorum-sensing inhibitors. A quorum-sensing system in staphylococci consists of the ribonucleic acid III (RNAIII)-activating peptide (RAP) and its target protein, target of RAP (TRAP).[5] Staphylococcal virulence is inhibited by RNAIII-inhibiting peptide (RIP), a linear heptapeptide resembling the N-terminal sequence of RAP that acts as an antagonist to TRAP. RIP inhibits the phosphorylation of TRAP, leading to reduced cell adhesion and suppression of toxin synthesis. Evidence also suggests that TRAP is involved in bacterial DNA protection from oxidative stress.[6] TRAP is conserved among staphylococcal species, hence RIP can theoretically suppress infections caused by any staphylococcal strain, including those resistant to methicillin or vancomycin. Synthetic RIP has been shown to be active in animal models of foreign body–associated infection,[7–9] and may have future utility as an alternative or adjunct to antimicrobials.

Bacteriophages are viruses that infect bacteria, and may have a role in controlling biofilm.[10] Bacteriophages may produce polysaccharide depolymerases that can hydrolyze polymeric substances in the biofilm matrix. The effect of bacteriophages on biofilms has been studied in vitro.[11,12] A bacteriophage was engineered to express a biofilm-degrading enzyme and simultaneously attack bacterial cells in the biofilm and the biofilm matrix.[13] The engineered enzymatic bacteriophage demonstrated greater in vitro efficacy than the nonenzymatic bacteriophage against biofilms. Use of bacteriophages to prevent colonization and subsequent infection may be applicable to urinary or intravascular catheters. In an in vitro model, pretreatment of hydrogel-coated silicone catheters with a single *Staphylococcus epidermidis* bacteriophage[14] or a cocktail of *Pseudomonas aeruginosa* bacteriophages[15] reduced biofilm formation.

ENHANCEMENT OF ANTIMICROBIAL ACTIVITY AGAINST BIOFILM BACTERIA

Electric current (EC) and ultrasound have been used adjunctively to antimicrobial agents to disrupt biofilms and treat infection. The bioelectric effect refers to the enhancement of antibacterial activity using EC. The proposed mechanisms include disruption of the biofilm matrix, membrane permeabilization and electrophoretic augmentation of antimicrobial transport, generation of oxygen as a result of electrolysis, and generation of potentiating oxidants.[16] Del Pozo and colleagues[17] described an in vitro model using biofilm-coated polytetrafluoroethylene coupons exposed to a continuous flow of fresh medium with or without antimicrobial agents and/or EC. A significant effect was found when vancomycin was used against methicillin-resistant *Staphylococcus aureus* (MRSA) biofilms and when daptomycin or erythromycin was used against *S epidermidis* biofilms in combination with EC. The bioelectric effect was not generalizable across microorganisms and antimicrobial agents. EC was also found to be active against bacterial biofilms when delivered without antimicrobials both in vitro[18] and in a rat model of foreign body–associated osteomyelitis,[19] an effect referred to as the electricidal effect.

The bioacoustic effect refers to the synergistic effect of ultrasound and antimicrobial agents in eradicating microbial biofilms. Simultaneous application of ultrasound and gentamicin to a polyethylene substrate reduced the viability of *P aeruginosa* biofilms,[20] achieved by using sufficiently low levels of ultrasonic power so that ultrasound by itself did not kill the bacteria. Lower-frequency ultrasound appears to be more effective than higher-frequency ultrasound in reducing bacterial viability within biofilms. The effect is also demonstrated in animal models of infection.[21] Several mechanisms have been proposed to explain the effect. Sonication increases transport of gentamicin across biofilms that normally block or slow antimicrobial transport when not exposed to ultrasound.[22] Low-frequency ultrasound increases outer membrane permeability of *P aeruginosa*,[23] and high-intensity focused ultrasound mechanically disrupts *Escherichia coli* biofilms grown on microscope slides.[24]

Another potential role of ultrasound is its application in combination with antimicrobial-impregnated cement. *E coli*, *P aeruginosa*, *S aureus*, and coagulase-negative staphylococci were tested in vitro using bone cements loaded with gentamicin or the combination of gentamicin and clindamycin. Application of pulsed ultrasound in combination with antibiotic release from bone cement yielded a reduction of both planktonic and biofilm bacterial viability compared with antibiotic release without application of ultrasound.[25] In a small animal study, bone cement disks loaded with gentamicin, on which *E coli* biofilms were grown, were implanted in rabbits. Application of ultrasound from 24 through 72 h after surgery resulted in a tendency toward improved efficacy of gentamicin.[26] The transducer was fixed to the rabbits using an acoustically conductive adhesive gel. Histopathological examination of skin showed no adverse effect associated with the applied pulsed ultrasound waves. Further data from in vitro and animal studies are necessary before applying these novel approaches to humans.

CATHETER-ASSOCIATED URINARY TRACT INFECTION

A catheterized patient with symptoms or signs referable to the urinary tract and significant bacteriuria is diagnosed as having a catheter-associated urinary tract infection (CAUTI). The exact relationship between asymptomatic bacteriuria and CAUTI remains unclear. Even though treatment of asymptomatic bacteriuria is generally not recommended (except in certain clinical conditions), it is plausible that preventing asymptomatic bacteriuria will decrease the incidence of symptomatic infection in catheterized patients.

Silver has broad-spectrum antimicrobial activity. In vitro studies show that coating urinary catheters with silver prevents adherence and growth of bacteria and inhibits biofilm formation.[27] A silver coating may be applied to the external and/or internal surface of a urinary catheter. The addition of hydrogel protects the mucosa and facilitates release of silver ions.[28] Hydrogel/silver-alloy catheters are latex-based or silicone-based. Silver oxide–coated catheters have been withdrawn from the market. Nitrofurazone-coated urinary catheters are silicone-based. Nitrofurazone is chemically related to nitrofurantoin. A disadvantage of this type of urinary catheter is that nitrofurazone is inactive against some uropathogens (eg, P aeruginosa). Minocycline/rifampin-impregnated urinary catheters are not available in the United States.

Table 1 summarizes the evidence from randomized and quasi-randomized trials on the efficacy of antimicrobial-coated catheters in preventing asymptomatic bacteriuria during short-term use.[29,30] The effect size varies among studies and the quality of evidence is considered fair. Data are conflicting, with some studies showing efficacy and others showing that silver coating is not effective. No published trial has directly compared different antimicrobial-coated catheters; hence it is unclear as to which type of catheter is most active. Development of symptomatic CAUTI, a clinically relevant end point, rather than development of bacteriuria, needs to be studied in well-designed, adequately powered, randomized clinical

Table 1
Evidence from randomized and quasi-randomized clinical trials on the efficacy of antimicrobial-coated urinary catheters in reducing the risk of asymptomatic bacteriuria during short-term (less than 30 days) use

Study[Ref.]	Silver Alloy–Impregnated Catheter	Nitrofurazone-Impregnated Catheter	Minocycline/Rifampin-Impregnated Catheter
Schumm and Lam,[29] 2008	<1 wk catheter use: RR 0.54 (95% CI 0.43–0.67)	<1 wk use: RR 0.52 (95% CI 0.34–0.78)	<1 wk use: RR 0.36 (95% CI 0.18–0.73)
	>1 wk use: RR 0.64 (95% CI 0.51–0.80)	>1 wk use: RR 0.31 (95% CI 0.06–1.66)	>1 wk use: RR 0.94 (95% CI 0.86–1.03)
Drekonja et al,[30] 2008	4 pre-1995 trials[a]: RRs 0.24–0.44 (median, 0.32) Absolute risk reduction 13%–32% (median, 28%) 5 post-1995 trials[a]: RRs 0.53–0.94 (median, 0.84) Absolute risk reduction 0.5%–5% (median, 2%)	4 trials[a]: RRs 0.08–0.68 (median, 0.45) Absolute risk reduction 3%–16% (median, 9.5%)	Not included

Risk ratio <1.0 favors antimicrobial-coated catheter use.
Abbreviations: CI, confidence interval; RR, risk ratio.
[a] Quantitative pooling of data not performed.

trials. The efficacy of antimicrobial-coated catheters also needs further study in chronically catheterized patients.

Another potential approach to prevent CAUTI is based on bacterial interference, the antagonism between bacteria during the process of surface colonization. Based on this concept, nonpathogenic organisms are used to compete with virulent bacteria.[31] In a pilot trial, patients with spinal cord injury and neurogenic bladder requiring indwelling (transurethral or suprapubic) or intermittent catheter drainage were randomized to this experimental treatment in comparison with placebo. In 21 patients, the bladder was inoculated with a nonpathogenic strain of E coli. In 7 patients the bladder was inoculated with normal saline. Patients colonized with the nonpathogenic E coli were significantly less likely than noncolonized patients to develop at least one episode of CAUTI during the 1-year follow-up period.[32]

CATHETER-ASSOCIATED BLOODSTREAM INFECTION

Central venous catheters are the most frequent source of nosocomial bloodstream infection. Accurate diagnosis is essential in the management of these infections. Intravascular catheter colonization is usually detected using the semiquantitative or roll-plate method, whereby a 5-cm catheter segment is rolled back and forth across the surface of a blood agar plate at least 4 times. The presence of 15 or more colony-forming units (CFU) after overnight incubation reflects catheter colonization. The roll-plate method samples the external catheter surface, and may miss organisms colonizing the internal surface. This limitation may be overcome by quantitative culture methods, whereby the catheter segment is flushed or immersed in a liquid and subsequently vortexed or sonicated.

A correlation between the frequency of concordant positive blood cultures and the number of organisms recovered from the vascular catheters after sonication has been reported.[33] Growth of more than 10^2 CFU from a catheter by quantitative (sonication) broth culture reflects catheter colonization. In a prospective, randomized, comparative study, the quantitative techniques of sonication or vortexing were not, however, superior to the semiquantitative technique for detecting catheter colonization.[34] Furthermore, among hematological patients with long-term tunneled catheters, sonication was not superior to the roll-plate method in diagnosing catheter colonization.[35] Given its simplicity and performance, the semiquantitative technique remains the most widely applied method in clinical laboratories.

Quantitative cultures drawn through the catheter and concomitantly by venipuncture from a peripheral vein or another catheter can be used for diagnostic purposes if the device is not removed. Quantitative cultures are obtained with the pour-plate technique or by using the lysis-centrifugation system. In the case of catheter infection, blood drawn through it typically shows a greater than fivefold increased concentration of organisms compared with blood drawn from a peripheral vein or another catheter. In a meta-analysis, the paired quantitative blood culture technique was found to be the most accurate among diagnostic methods not necessitating catheter removal.[36] However, quantitative blood cultures are labor intensive and expensive.

An alternative technique is based on the differential time to positivity of blood cultures. Positivity in a blood culture drawn from the catheter more than 2 hours before positivity of a culture drawn from a peripheral vein is highly predictive of catheter-associated bloodstream infection (CABSI). In a prospective study, the sensitivity and specificity of the method in patients with short-term catheters (<30 days) were 81% and 92%, respectively; for those with long-term catheters (≥30 days), differential time to positivity had a sensitivity of 93% and a specificity of 75%.[37] In patients with multilumen catheters, when blood cultures are drawn to diagnose CABSI these should be collected through all catheter lumens.[38]

In terms of CABSI prevention, use of antiseptic/antimicrobial-impregnated catheters is recommended if infection rates are elevated despite use of maximal sterile barrier precautions, and skin antisepsis with chlorhexidine during insertion.[39] Evidence from a meta-analysis is summarized in **Table 2**.[40] Antiseptic catheters are coated with chlorhexidine and sulfadiazine silver. First-generation catheters are coated only on the external surface, whereas second-generation catheters are coated on both the external and internal surfaces. First-generation catheters reduced the risk for CABSI compared with standard noncoated catheters. Second-generation catheters have demonstrated a reduction in catheter colonization, but the studies were underpowered to show a difference in CABSI.[41–43] The silver iontophoretic catheter is impregnated with silver, platinum, and carbon, and releases silver ions topically. One study showed a reduction in the incidence of catheter colonization and CABSI,[44] but others found no difference.[45,46]

The antimicrobial-coated catheter approved by the Food and Drug Administration is impregnated with minocycline and rifampin on both internal and external surfaces. In a prospective, randomized clinical trial, use of minocycline/rifampin-impregnated catheters was associated with a lower rate of CABSI than first-generation chlorhexidine/silver-impregnated catheters (0.3% vs 3.4%, $P<.002$).[47] A comparison with second-generation chlorhexidine/silver-impregnated catheters has not been conducted. In a study among cancer patients, long-term nontunneled silicone catheters impregnated with minocycline/rifampin were also efficacious in reducing CABSI.[48] No emergence of antimicrobial resistance was detected in these studies.

Use of catheter lock solutions is another strategy to prevent biofilm formation and/or eradicate established biofilm. Using this technique, parenteral antimicrobials or antiseptics are infused into the catheter hub and allowed to dwell at supratherapeutic concentrations. The antimicrobial or antiseptic (eg, alcohol, taurolidine, trisodium citrate) is usually combined with an anticoagulant, such as heparin or ethylenediamine tetra-acetic acid. Most studies focus on patients at high risk for CABSI. Antimicrobial lock solutions reduce the risk of CABSI in patients undergoing hemodialysis[49] and in immunocompromised pediatric patients.[50] Similarly, alcohol lock solution decreases the risk of infection among immunosuppressed hematology patients.[51] In general, prophylactic administration of lock solution is recommended for patients with

Table 2
Evidence from randomized controlled trials on the efficacy of antimicrobial-coated central venous catheters in reducing the risk of catheter colonization and catheter-associated bloodstream infection

Catheter Type	Central Venous Catheter Colonization	Catheter-Associated Bloodstream Infection
First-generation chlorhexidine/silver sulfadiazine	0.51 (0.42–0.61)	0.68 (0.47–0.98)
Second-generation chlorhexidine/silver sulfadiazine	0.39 (0.25–0.60)	0.47 (0.20–1.10)
Silver iontophoretic	0.84 (0.60–1.16)	1.98 (0.40–9.95)
Minocycline/rifampin	0.39 (0.27–0.55)	0.29 (0.16–0.52)

Values represent pooled odds ratios (95% confidence interval). Odds ratio <1.0 favors antimicrobial-coated catheter use.
Data from Casey AL, Mermel LA, Nightingale P, et al. Antimicrobial central venous catheters in adults: a systematic review and meta-analysis. Lancet Infect Dis 2008;8(12):763–76.

long-term catheters who have a history of multiple infections despite maximal adherence to aseptic techniques.[39] Antibiotic-lock therapy in conjunction with systemic antimicrobial therapy is used in patients with CABSI involving long-term catheters with no signs of exit site or tunnel infection for whom catheter salvage is the goal.[52]

INFECTION ASSOCIATED WITH ORTHOPEDIC IMPLANTS

Orthopedic implants include prosthetic joints, spine implants, fracture-fixation devices, pins, screws, and plates, as well as intramedullary nails. The microbiological diagnosis of orthopedic implant–associated infection is traditionally based on culture of synovial fluid and surgically obtained peri-implant tissue. For hip and knee prosthetic joint infection (PJI), the collection of 5 or 6 tissue specimens has been recommended.[53] An alternative diagnostic approach is directed toward detecting biofilm bacteria that attach to the surface of the implant. Using this method, the implant is placed in a container with sterile saline, vortexed, and sonicated in an ultrasonic bath. This procedure causes biofilm bacteria to dislodge and disaggregate. Aliquots of the sonicate fluid are then cultured; growth in significant quantity correlates with implant infection.

Culture of samples obtained by sonication is more sensitive than conventional periprosthetic tissue culture for the diagnosis of infection associated with hip or knee,[54] shoulder,[55] and spine implants (**Table 3**).[56] For prosthetic elbow infection, culture of the implant using sonication is at least as sensitive as periprosthetic tissue culture.[57] Notably for hip or knee infection, the sensitivity of sonicate culture was similar to tissue culture if 5 or more tissue specimens were cultured. An added benefit is that sonicate cultures have a shorter time to positivity than tissue cultures.[58]

Molecular techniques are attractive tools for the diagnosis of PJI. Broad-range polymerase chain reaction (PCR) may be applied (eg, amplifying the 16S ribosomal RNA gene). For organism identification, amplified product analysis (eg, by sequencing) is needed. Multiplex PCR may be used to amplify genomic DNA using multiple primers, allowing direct species identification. PCR has been evaluated in synovial fluid, periprosthetic tissue, and most recently sonicate fluid. In the authors' experience, *Propionibacterium acnes* and *Staphylococcus* spp account for most positive sonicate fluid cultures among subjects with prosthetic shoulder infection; these cases can be detected by PCR of sonicate fluid.[55]

In a study of 69 orthopedic implants, the sensitivity of PCR of sonicate fluid was similar to that of the combined cultures of periprosthetic tissue and sonicate fluid

Table 3
Comparison of sonicate fluid and periprosthetic tissue culture for the diagnosis of infection associated with orthopedic implants

Implant Type		Sonicate Fluid	Periprosthetic Tissue	P Value	Reference
Prosthetic hip/knee joint	Sensitivity	78.5%	60.8%	<0.001	Trampuz et al,[54] 2007
	Specificity	98.8%	99.2%		
Prosthetic shoulder joint	Sensitivity	66.7%	54.5%	0.046	Piper et al,[55] 2009
	Specificity	98.0%	95.1%		
Prosthetic elbow joint	Sensitivity	89%	55%	0.18	Vergidis et al,[57] 2011
	Specificity	100%	93%		
Spine implant	Sensitivity	91%	73%	0.046	Sampedro et al,[56] 2010
	Specificity	97%	93%		

(92.3% vs 92.9%).[59] In another study of 37 cases of PJI, the causative organisms were identified in periprosthetic tissue culture in 65% of cases, in sonication fluid culture in 62%, and by multiplex PCR in 78%.[60] The approach is particularly useful in those receiving preoperative antibiotics. In addition, molecular approaches may be more rapid than culture-based diagnostics. Molecular techniques may, however, yield false-positive results. In a prospective study of patients undergoing revision total hip or knee arthroplasty because of prosthesis failure, synovial fluid was collected intraoperatively. Twelve joints (13%) were found to be infected, but PCR was positive in 32 cases.[61] The positive predictive value was only 34%. The clinical significance of detection of microbial nucleic acid in not obviously infected implants and/or representing organisms not traditionally associated with PJI needs further study.

Inflammatory serum markers used to identify PJI preoperatively include white blood cell (WBC) count, erythrocyte sedimentation rate (ESR), and C-reactive protein (CRP). Novel diagnostic markers include interleukin (IL)-6, procalcitonin, and tumor necrosis factor α. In a meta-analysis of 30 studies including 3909 revision total hip or knee arthroplasties, IL-6 and CRP level had a higher diagnostic odds ratio than ESR and WBC count in discriminating infectious from noninfectious causes of prosthesis failure.[62] Only 3 studies of IL-6 were included, and the investigators concluded that further investigation is warranted. High serum IgM antibody levels to staphylococcal slime polysaccharide antigens may aid in the detection of the immune response elicited by biofilm colonization. An enzyme-linked immunosorbent assay has been developed and tested in a single study of 90 patients. The assay demonstrated a sensitivity of 89.7% and a specificity of 95.1% in detecting PJI caused by S aureus and/or coagulase-negative staphylococci.[63] For patients with abnormal ESR and/or CRP, joint aspiration should be performed. Aspirated fluid should be sent for WBC count with differential and culture. The diagnostic utility of novel synovial fluid biomarkers (eg, IL-1β, granulocyte-colony stimulating factor, IL-6, CRP) is being evaluated.[64]

It is arguable that orthopedic implant infections are best prevented. Most prosthetic joint infections likely originate from implant contamination at implantation.[65] Preoperative intravenous antimicrobial prophylaxis is recommended for patients undergoing primary arthroplasty. Use of antibiotic-impregnated bone cement is another strategy, but is not universally applied in primary arthroplasty. In a study using the Norwegian Arthroplasty Register, the risk of subsequent revision hip arthroplasty (because of aseptic failure or infection) was lowest when antibiotic prophylaxis was given both systemically and in the cement.[66] Concerns regarding the prophylactic use of antibiotic-impregnated cement include selection of antimicrobial resistance, allergic reactions, compromise of cement mechanical properties, and cost.

Postoperatively, bacteremia from any source may lead to hematogenous seeding and infection of the prosthetic implant. The American Academy of Orthopaedic Surgeons has issued an information statement favoring antimicrobial prophylaxis in patients with prosthetic joints undergoing dental, gastrointestinal, genitourinary, or other invasive procedures. Nonetheless, the available evidence does not support this recommendation. In a prospective case-control study, dental procedures were not associated with an increased risk of prosthetic knee or hip infection.[67] Furthermore, prophylactic antimicrobials prior to dental procedures were not associated with a decreased risk of infection.

Based on the concept of quorum-sensing signaling systems that coordinate biological activity, development of a microelectromechanical systems–type biosensing device has been proposed.[68] This device would function as an intelligent implant, detecting bacterial communication systems associated with quorum sensing. On intercepting bacterial signals, the biosensor would send a signal to gated reservoirs that would release compounds inhibitory to biofilm formation, and local antibiotics that would eradicate planktonic bacteria in proximity to the implant before establishment of biofilm.

INFECTION OF CARDIOVASCULAR IMPLANTABLE ELECTRONIC DEVICES

CIEDs include pacemakers, implantable cardioverter-defibrillators, and cardiac resynchronization therapy devices. Microbiological diagnosis of CIED infections is based on organism isolation from the pocket site, the infected generator, the lead, or the bloodstream. The sensitivity of tissue culture of the fibrous capsule is higher than that of swab culture from the deep pocket site.[69] The explanted generator and lead tips can also be cultured. Sonication of the explanted device may aid in the diagnosis of CIED infection. However, it remains unclear whether this approach provides value beyond conventional strategies. A study of generators infected in vitro with a biofilm-producing strain of MRSA demonstrated that the use of vortexing, sonication, and incubation of the device in trypticase soy broth yielded similar results to broth incubation alone.[70] The sonication technique has been evaluated in a small clinical study.[71] Sonicate fluid cultures demonstrated a diagnostic yield that was comparable to that of tissue cultures. Both were superior to swab cultures. The combined use of sonication, tissue, blood, and lead-tip cultures resulted in detection of bacteria in all patients with pocket infections.

The significance of bacteria colonizing CIEDs is not entirely clear. Such bacteria may represent asymptomatic colonization or subclinical infection. In a study of patients with explanted cardiac devices without clinical signs of infection, bacteria were detected in 38% of sonicate fluid and 27% of conventional generator pocket swab cultures.[72] P acnes and coagulase-negative staphylococci, both common skin commensals, were the most frequently isolated bacteria. In a similar study of 108 asymptomatic patients, 47% demonstrated bacterial DNA on devices replaced for battery depletion.[73]

Early CIED infections generally result from wound contamination at the time of placement, and preventive strategies have been developed to reduce this risk. Perioperative antibiotic prophylaxis can reduce the incidence of CIED infection, as was shown in a randomized, double-blind, controlled trial of single-dose cefazolin.[74] Despite prophylactic measures, the number of infections continues to increase out of proportion to implantation rates,[75] probably due to the increasing complexity of cases. Novel preventive approaches, such as local antimicrobial delivery methods, are needed. In a multicenter study of 624 consecutive procedures, use of a polypropylene mesh envelope releasing minocycline and rifampin in the generator pocket was associated with a low infection rate at a mean follow-up of 1.9 months.[76] This novel technique needs additional study in a prospective randomized fashion.

SUMMARY

The pathogenesis of device-associated infections relates to bacteria that attach to and grow on surfaces in complex communities. Biofilm bacteria are severalfold more resistant to antimicrobial agents in comparison with planktonic counterparts. Novel diagnostic approaches directed toward detecting biofilm bacteria have been developed. Innovative approaches to prevention and treatment now being evaluated include the use of antisense molecules, quorum-sensing inhibitors, bacteriophages that hydrolyze biofilm matrix, and bacterial interference. EC and ultrasound may be used in the future adjunctively to antimicrobials to disrupt biofilms and treat infection, and EC alone may be useful to prevent and/or treat biofilm-associated infections.

REFERENCES

1. del Pozo JL, Patel R. The challenge of treating biofilm-associated bacterial infections. Clin Pharmacol Ther 2007;82(2):204–9.
2. Costerton WJ, Montanaro L, Balaban N, et al. Prospecting gene therapy of implant infections. Int J Artif Organs 2009;32(9):689–95.
3. Speziale P, Pietrocola G, Rindi S, et al. Structural and functional role of *Staphylococcus aureus* surface components recognizing adhesive matrix molecules of the host. Future Microbiol 2009;4(10):1337–52.
4. O'Gara JP. *ica* and beyond: biofilm mechanisms and regulation in *Staphylococcus epidermidis* and *Staphylococcus aureus.* FEMS Microbiol Lett 2007; 270(2):179–88.
5. Balaban N, Stoodley P, Fux CA, et al. Prevention of staphylococcal biofilm-associated infections by the quorum sensing inhibitor RIP. Clin Orthop Relat Res 2005;437:48–54.
6. Kiran MD, Balaban N. TRAP plays a role in stress response in *Staphylococcus aureus.* Int J Artif Organs 2009;32(9):592–9.
7. Anguita-Alonso P, Giacometti A, Cirioni O, et al. RNAIII-inhibiting-peptide-loaded polymethylmethacrylate prevents in vivo *Staphylococcus aureus* biofilm formation. Antimicrob Agents Chemother 2007;51(7):2594–6.
8. Balaban N, Cirioni O, Giacometti A, et al. Treatment of *Staphylococcus aureus* biofilm infection by the quorum-sensing inhibitor RIP. Antimicrob Agents Chemother 2007;51(6):2226–9.
9. Cirioni O, Ghiselli R, Minardi D, et al. RNAIII-inhibiting peptide affects biofilm formation in a rat model of staphylococcal ureteral stent infection. Antimicrob Agents Chemother 2007;51(12):4518–20.
10. Donlan RM. Preventing biofilms of clinically relevant organisms using bacteriophage. Trends Microbiol 2009;17(2):66–72.
11. Cerca N, Oliveira R, Azeredo J. Susceptibility of *Staphylococcus epidermidis* planktonic cells and biofilms to the lytic action of staphylococcus bacteriophage K. Lett Appl Microbiol 2007;45(3):313–7.
12. Sharma M, Ryu JH, Beuchat LR. Inactivation of *Escherichia coli* O157:H7 in biofilm on stainless steel by treatment with an alkaline cleaner and a bacteriophage. J Appl Microbiol 2005;99(3):449–59.
13. Lu TK, Collins JJ. Dispersing biofilms with engineered enzymatic bacteriophage. Proc Natl Acad Sci U S A 2007;104(27):11197–202.
14. Curtin JJ, Donlan RM. Using bacteriophages to reduce formation of catheter-associated biofilms by *Staphylococcus epidermidis.* Antimicrob Agents Chemother 2006;50(4):1268–75.
15. Fu W, Forster T, Mayer O, et al. Bacteriophage cocktail for the prevention of biofilm formation by *Pseudomonas aeruginosa* on catheters in an in vitro model system. Antimicrob Agents Chemother 2010;54(1):397–404.
16. Del Pozo JL, Rouse MS, Patel R. Bioelectric effect and bacterial biofilms. A systematic review. Int J Artif Organs 2008;31(9):786–95.
17. del Pozo JL, Rouse MS, Mandrekar JN, et al. Effect of electrical current on the activities of antimicrobial agents against *Pseudomonas aeruginosa,*

Staphylococcus aureus, and *Staphylococcus epidermidis* biofilms. Antimicrob Agents Chemother 2009;53(1):35–40.

18. del Pozo JL, Rouse MS, Mandrekar JN, et al. The electricidal effect: reduction of *Staphylococcus* and *Pseudomonas* biofilms by prolonged exposure to low-intensity electrical current. Antimicrob Agents Chemother 2009;53(1):41–5.

19. Del Pozo JL, Rouse MS, Euba G, et al. The electricidal effect is active in an experimental model of *Staphylococcus epidermidis* chronic foreign body osteomyelitis. Antimicrob Agents Chemother 2009;53(10):4064–8.

20. Qian Z, Sagers RD, Pitt WG. The effect of ultrasonic frequency upon enhanced killing of *P. aeruginosa* biofilms. Ann Biomed Eng 1997;25(1):69–76.

21. Rediske AM, Roeder BL, Nelson JL, et al. Pulsed ultrasound enhances the killing of *Escherichia coli* biofilms by aminoglycoside antibiotics in vivo. Antimicrob Agents Chemother 2000;44(3):771–2.

22. Carmen JC, Nelson JL, Beckstead BL, et al. Ultrasonic-enhanced gentamicin transport through colony biofilms of *Pseudomonas aeruginosa* and *Escherichia coli*. J Infect Chemother 2004;10(4):193–9.

23. Runyan CM, Carmen JC, Beckstead BL, et al. Low-frequency ultrasound increases outer membrane permeability of *Pseudomonas aeruginosa*. J Gen Appl Microbiol 2006;52(5):295–301.

24. Bigelow TA, Northagen T, Hill TM, et al. The destruction of *Escherichia coli* biofilms using high-intensity focused ultrasound. Ultrasound Med Biol 2009;35(6): 1026–31.

25. Ensing GT, Neut D, van Horn JR, et al. The combination of ultrasound with antibiotics released from bone cement decreases the viability of planktonic and biofilm bacteria: An in vitro study with clinical strains. J Antimicrob Chemother 2006; 58(6):1287–90.

26. Ensing GT, Roeder BL, Nelson JL, et al. Effect of pulsed ultrasound in combination with gentamicin on bacterial viability in biofilms on bone cements in vivo. J Appl Microbiol 2005;99(3):443–8.

27. Ahearn DG, Grace DT, Jennings MJ, et al. Effects of hydrogel/silver coatings on in vitro adhesion to catheters of bacteria associated with urinary tract infections. Curr Microbiol 2000;41(2):120–5.

28. Davenport K, Keeley FX. Evidence for the use of silver-alloy-coated urethral catheters. J Hosp Infect 2005;60(4):298–303.

29. Schumm K, Lam TB. Types of urethral catheters for management of short-term voiding problems in hospitalised adults. Cochrane Database Syst Rev 2008;2:CD004013.

30. Drekonja DM, Kuskowski MA, Wilt TJ, et al. Antimicrobial urinary catheters: a systematic review. Expert Rev Med Devices 2008;5(4):495–506.

31. Trautner BW, Hull RA, Darouiche RO. *Escherichia coli* 83972 inhibits catheter adherence by a broad spectrum of uropathogens. Urology 2003;61(5):1059–62.

32. Darouiche RO, Thornby JI, Cerra-Stewart C, et al. Bacterial interference for prevention of urinary tract infection: A prospective, randomized, placebo-controlled, double-blind pilot trial. Clin Infect Dis 2005;41(10):1531–4.

33. Sherertz RJ, Raad II, Belani A, et al. Three-year experience with sonicated vascular catheter cultures in a clinical microbiology laboratory. J Clin Microbiol 1990;28(1):76–82.

34. Bouza E, Alvarado N, Alcala L, et al. A prospective, randomized, and comparative study of 3 different methods for the diagnosis of intravascular catheter colonization. Clin Infect Dis 2005;40(8):1096–100.

35. Slobbe L, El Barzouhi A, Boersma E, et al. Comparison of the roll plate method to the sonication method to diagnose catheter colonization and bacteremia in

patients with long-term tunnelled catheters: a randomized prospective study. J Clin Microbiol 2009;47(4):885–8.

36. Safdar N, Fine JP, Maki DG. Meta-analysis: methods for diagnosing intravascular device-related bloodstream infection. Ann Intern Med 2005;142(6):451–66.

37. Raad I, Hanna HA, Alakech B, et al. Differential time to positivity: a useful method for diagnosing catheter-related bloodstream infections. Ann Intern Med 2004; 140(1):18–25.

38. Guembe M, Rodriguez-Creixems M, Sanchez-Carrillo C, et al. How many lumens should be cultured in the conservative diagnosis of catheter-related bloodstream infections? Clin Infect Dis 2010;50(12):1575–9.

39. O'Grady NP, Alexander M, Burns LA, et al. Guidelines for the prevention of intravascular catheter-related infections. Clin Infect Dis 2011;52(9):e162–93.

40. Casey AL, Mermel LA, Nightingale P, et al. Antimicrobial central venous catheters in adults: a systematic review and meta-analysis. Lancet Infect Dis 2008;8(12): 763–76.

41. Brun-Buisson C, Doyon F, Sollet JP, et al. Prevention of intravascular catheter-related infection with newer chlorhexidine-silver sulfadiazine-coated catheters: a randomized controlled trial. Intensive Care Med 2004;30(5):837–43.

42. Ostendorf T, Meinhold A, Harter C, et al. Chlorhexidine and silver-sulfadiazine coated central venous catheters in haematological patients—a double-blind, randomised, prospective, controlled trial. Support Care Cancer 2005;13(12): 993–1000.

43. Rupp ME, Lisco SJ, Lipsett PA, et al. Effect of a second-generation venous catheter impregnated with chlorhexidine and silver sulfadiazine on central catheter-related infections: a randomized, controlled trial. Ann Intern Med 2005; 143(8):570–80.

44. Corral L, Nolla-Salas M, Ibanez-Nolla J, et al. A prospective, randomized study in critically ill patients using the Oligon Vantex catheter. J Hosp Infect 2003;55(3): 212–9.

45. Hagau N, Studnicska D, Gavrus RL, et al. Central venous catheter colonization and catheter-related bloodstream infections in critically ill patients: a comparison between standard and silver-integrated catheters. Eur J Anaesthesiol 2009;26(9): 752–8.

46. Bong JJ, Kite P, Wilco MH, et al. Prevention of catheter related bloodstream infection by silver iontophoretic central venous catheters: a randomised controlled trial. J Clin Pathol 2003;56(10):731–5.

47. Darouiche RO, Raad II, Heard SO, et al. A comparison of two antimicrobial-impregnated central venous catheters. Catheter Study Group. N Engl J Med 1999;340(1):1–8.

48. Hanna H, Benjamin R, Chatzinikolaou I, et al. Long-term silicone central venous catheters impregnated with minocycline and rifampin decrease rates of catheter-related bloodstream infection in cancer patients: a prospective randomized clinical trial. J Clin Oncol 2004;22(15):3163–71.

49. Yahav D, Rozen-Zvi B, Gafter-Gvili A, et al. Antimicrobial lock solutions for the prevention of infections associated with intravascular catheters in patients undergoing hemodialysis: systematic review and meta-analysis of randomized, controlled trials. Clin Infect Dis 2008;47(1):83–93.

50. Henrickson KJ, Axtell RA, Hoover SM, et al. Prevention of central venous catheter-related infections and thrombotic events in immunocompromised children by the use of vancomycin/ciprofloxacin/heparin flush solution: a randomized, multicenter, double-blind trial. J Clin Oncol 2000;18(6):1269–78.

51. Sanders J, Pithie A, Ganly P, et al. A prospective double-blind randomized trial comparing intraluminal ethanol with heparinized saline for the prevention of catheter-associated bloodstream infection in immunosuppressed haematology patients. J Antimicrob Chemother 2008;62(4):809–15.
52. Fortun J, Grill F, Martin-Davila P, et al. Treatment of long-term intravascular catheter-related bacteraemia with antibiotic-lock therapy. J Antimicrob Chemother 2006;58(4):816–21.
53. Atkins BL, Athanasou N, Deeks JJ, et al. Prospective evaluation of criteria for microbiological diagnosis of prosthetic-joint infection at revision arthroplasty. The OSIRIS Collaborative Study Group. J Clin Microbiol 1998;36(10):2932–9.
54. Trampuz A, Piper KE, Jacobson MJ, et al. Sonication of removed hip and knee prostheses for diagnosis of infection. N Engl J Med 2007;357(7):654–63.
55. Piper KE, Jacobson MJ, Cofield RH, et al. Microbiologic diagnosis of prosthetic shoulder infection by use of implant sonication. J Clin Microbiol 2009;47(6): 1878–84.
56. Sampedro MF, Huddleston PM, Piper KE, et al. A biofilm approach to detect bacteria on removed spinal implants. Spine 2010;35(12):1218–24.
57. Vergidis P, Greenwood-Quaintance KE, Sanchez-Sotelo, et al. Implant sonication for the diagnosis of prosthetic elbow infection. J Shoulder Elbow Surg (in press).
58. Dailey A, Nyre L, Piper K, et al. Hip or knee prosthesis sonicate cultures have a shorter time to positivity compared to periprosthetic tissue cultures. 49th Interscience Conference on Antimicrobial Agents and Chemotherapy. San Francisco (CA), September 12–15, 2009.
59. Dora C, Altwegg M, Gerber C, et al. Evaluation of conventional microbiological procedures and molecular genetic techniques for diagnosis of infections in patients with implanted orthopedic devices. J Clin Microbiol 2008;46(2):824–5.
60. Achermann Y, Vogt M, Leunig M, et al. Improved diagnosis of periprosthetic joint infection by multiplex PCR of sonication fluid from removed implants. J Clin Microbiol 2010;48(4):1208–14.
61. Panousis K, Grigoris P, Butcher I, et al. Poor predictive value of broad-range PCR for the detection of arthroplasty infection in 92 cases. Acta Orthop 2005;76(3):341–6.
62. Berbari E, Mabry T, Tsaras G, et al. Inflammatory blood laboratory levels as markers of prosthetic joint infection: a systematic review and meta-analysis. J Bone Joint Surg Am 2010;92(11):2102–9.
63. Artini M, Romano C, Manzoli L, et al. Staphylococcal IgM enzyme-linked immunosorbent assay for diagnosis of periprosthetic joint infections. J Clin Microbiol 2011;49(1):423–5.
64. Deirmengian C, Hallab N, Tarabishy A, et al. Synovial fluid biomarkers for periprosthetic infection. Clin Orthop Relat Res 2010;468(8):2017–23.
65. Jacovides CL, Parvizi J, Adeli B, et al. Molecular markers for diagnosis of periprosthetic joint infection. J Arthroplasty 2011;26(6 Suppl):99–103.
66. Engesaeter LB, Lie SA, Espehaug B, et al. Antibiotic prophylaxis in total hip arthroplasty: effects of antibiotic prophylaxis systemically and in bone cement on the revision rate of 22,170 primary hip replacements followed 0-14 years in the Norwegian Arthroplasty Register. Acta Orthop Scand 2003;74(6):644–51.
67. Berbari EF, Osmon DR, Carr A, et al. Dental procedures as risk factors for prosthetic hip or knee infection: a hospital-based prospective case-control study. Clin Infect Dis 2010;50(1):8–16.
68. Ehrlich GD, Stoodley P, Kathju S, et al. Engineering approaches for the detection and control of orthopaedic biofilm infections. Clin Orthop Relat Res 2005;(437): 59–66.

69. Dy Chua J, Abdul-Karim A, Mawhorter S, et al. The role of swab and tissue culture in the diagnosis of implantable cardiac device infection. Pacing Clin Electrophysiol 2005;28(12):1276–81.
70. Viola GM, Mansouri MD, Nasir N Jr, et al. Incubation alone is adequate as a culturing technique for cardiac rhythm management devices. J Clin Microbiol 2009;47(12):4168–70.
71. Mason PK, Dimarco JP, Ferguson JD, et al. Sonication of explanted cardiac rhythm management devices for the diagnosis of pocket infections and asymptomatic bacterial colonization. Pacing Clin Electrophysiol 2011;34(2):143–9.
72. Rohacek M, Weisser M, Kobza R, et al. Bacterial colonization and infection of electrophysiological cardiac devices detected with sonication and swab culture. Circulation 2010;121(15):1691–7.
73. Pichlmaier M, Marwitz V, Kuhn C, et al. High prevalence of asymptomatic bacterial colonization of rhythm management devices. Europace 2008;10(9):1067–72.
74. de Oliveira JC, Martinelli M, Nishioka SA, et al. Efficacy of antibiotic prophylaxis before the implantation of pacemakers and cardioverter-defibrillators: results of a large, prospective, randomized, double-blinded, placebo-controlled trial. Circ Arrhythm Electrophysiol 2009;2(1):29–34.
75. Voigt A, Shalaby A, Saba S. Continued rise in rates of cardiovascular implantable electronic device infections in the United States: temporal trends and causative insights. Pacing Clin Electrophysiol 2010;33(4):414–9.
76. Bloom HL, Constantin L, Dan D, et al. Implantation success and infection in cardiovascular implantable electronic device procedures utilizing an antibacterial envelope. Pacing Clin Electrophysiol 2011;34(2):133–42.

Index

Note: Page numbers of article titles are in **boldface** type.

A

Antimicrobial agents
    in CIED infection management, 65–68
    in urinary catheter–associated infection prevention, 24
    in VGIs prevention, 52
    in VRIs management, 94–95
Aortic grafts
    in VGIs prevention, 46–49
Arteriovenous hemodialysis grafts ((AVHGs))
    VGIs in, 41
AVHGs. *See* Arteriovenous hemodialysis grafts (AVHGs)

B

Bacteremia
    S. aureus
        management of
            in CIED infection management, 63–64
Bacteriuria
    catheter-acquired, 14
    in urinary catheter–associated infections, 14
Biofilm bacteria
    formation of
        antimicrobial activity against, 175
        medical device–associated infections related to
            prevention of, 174–175
Breast implant(s)
    placement of, 111
    types of, 112
Breast implant infections, **111–125**
    costs related to, 112
    diagnosis of, 117
    epidemiology of, 112
    management of, 118–119
    microbiology of, 114–117
    pathogenesis of, 114–117
    prevention of, 119–121
    risk factors for, 112–114
Bundles
    in VRIs prevention, 96

Infect Dis Clin N Am 26 (2012) 187–193
doi:10.1016/S0891-5520(11)00108-5
0891-5520/12/$ – see front matter © 2012 Elsevier Inc. All rights reserved.

id.theclinics.com

Moving?

Make sure your subscription moves with you!

To notify us of your new address, find your **Clinics Account Number** (located on your mailing label above your name), and contact customer service at:

Email: journalscustomerservice-usa@elsevier.com

800-654-2452 (subscribers in the U.S. & Canada)
314-447-8871 (subscribers outside of the U.S. & Canada)

Fax number: 314-447-8029

Elsevier Health Sciences Division
Subscription Customer Service
3251 Riverport Lane
Maryland Heights, MO 63043

*To ensure uninterrupted delivery of your subscription, please notify us at least 4 weeks in advance of move.

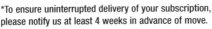

Printed and bound by CPI Group (UK) Ltd, Croydon, CR0 4YY

15/10/2024

01774217-0001